Boost Your Health

Strategies for strengthening your body health with Foods, Herbs and Stress Management

By: Melvin Madron

The trademarks that are used are without any consent, and the publication of the trademark is without permission or backing by the trademark owner. All trademarks and brands within this book are for clarifying purposes only and are the owned by the owners themselves, not affiliated with this document.

Table of Content

Introduction

Successful exploration of how one should live to the fullest is nothing less than an arcane. Therefore, a well-versed terminology is health regarding a day to day situation in a person's life, which evolves regarding the physical, emotional, or mental condition round the clock. The idea behind it is boosting your immunity. And the ability to do so requires several measures for several reasons. A person's immune system is precisely a system that functions well with a balanced harmony. Thus there are significant links of enhancing lifestyle through boosting physical nature with the focus on healthy living. The question that strikes the thoughts is; can health be improved? There are so many factors that are responsible in staying healthy. In turn, good health can decrease your risk of developing certain conditions. These include heart disease, stroke, some cancers, and injuries. It is important to learn what a person can do to maintain his/her and one's family's health. It is normal to consider a casual way of living first hand, but if unhealthy measures are neglected, then it is categorized as being unhealthy. There are people who are attentive towards being healthy; each move they make completely focuses on how to boost their health. The people fortunate enough to live a healthy life, by time, develops the habits. The ideal use of resources and managing situations enables them to make the right decisions. This sort of approach of ceasing timely decisions and resource utilization helps you with healthy living and discovering new and proven ways to boost health for a healthy life.

An unhealthy lifestyle is considered to be something that destroys the flavors of nature. Talking about the very nature and beginning, it usually starts with the initial stages of human anatomy and the related life cycle process.

You simply just cannot assume thinking about a case where a sudden average declines take place in later stages of life.

Learning about the demographics and life cycle process regardless of which part of the world is talked about, health hazards originate from the birth process and binds itself to the six feet under. The factors influencing varies from food to psychological factors, which have the most impact in general. When looking for a possible solution, it is important to take the calculated initiatives endorsed all over the globe.

There are things related to society that most of the time, are responsible for the worst possible health hazards. There are numerous social issues and problems that directly or indirectly creates a mess of a healthy life. It is to be considered as the negativity of the mind resulting from stress, results in unhealthy outcomes. Being a victim of a bad health condition say; the obesity, is not usually occurring from bad food and nutrition factor, but there is the stress that do play a vital role. Such a stress factor is indulged in a number of social determinants having bad experiences and negative interactions with individuals and events. These issues are legitimately effective by all means and could be tackled if not ignored with respect to their influence on healthy living.

It is a delight as we speak that there are so many ways we can follow in our routine which are useful to overcome the problem of unhealthiness and in fact, help us to boost our health. The factors related to the maximization of health standards can be dealt with by adding healthy foods in our life, adding proper meal plans, and a complete understanding of diet varieties with related pros and cons, adding more to it by fighting social issues to manage stress by using different techniques. Utilizing the right types of foods and greens makes you resilient to fight bad health. Similarly, managing stress can help you to overcome the social issues and adding up a successful and healthy lifestyle, and connect with people and the very moments by enjoying them to the fullest.

This book stores all the important information that explains the origins and solutions regarding how to boost your health, what associated factors it has, what sort of difference it can make and in-depth analysis of demerits related to human life cycle and the social determinants, how health could be boosted up with the use of foods and herbs and planning appropriate diet plans, observing your routine life which can be helpful to manage stress, as well as how to take ideal actions for the positive results in order to enjoy the healthy life and make your future better.

Chapter 1: Understanding Healthy life

A detailed understanding of health is discussed in this chapter. Health is the lifeline of our body, and it is impossible to understand it without the in-depth knowledge of a Healthy life. Along with it, we will discuss the associated factors and influences it can make in our routine. The health and wellness have gone through somewhat of a revolution in the recent past. Junk food and drinks have somehow taken the backseat, as now consumers want relatively healthier products.

According to various health studies, it has been found that in recent years people have lived a healthier lifestyle compared to the past decades, and it is said that people have made significant changes to improve their overall health and well-being.

Is this healthy life a mere fad? A theme to pass? We've reached 2020 and feel it's safe to say that the healthy living trend is here to stay. People are much more aware than ever compared to what they eat and how much exercise they regularly get. A fundamental shift in demand for healthy food has been witnessed by the food industry alone, and its rapid growth shows no signs of slowing down.

There is also a steady rise in social media influencers on stress management, fitness preparation, and clean eating, which use their platforms to always put the message of healthy living before us. Healthy living, though, is not just a phenomenon, it's a way of life that we should all follow in the interests of our health.

1.1 Basic Introduction to Health

What is health?

Health is not particularly just an absence of illness, but an overall state of well-being, indicating that the term health applies to a state of complete emotional and physical well-being. Quick wellness details include some primary health concerns. Some important information provided here states.

• Health can be described in detail as physical, mental, and social well-being and a life-long resource.

• This applies not only to the lack of sickness but also to the ability to recover and recover from disease and other problems.

• Good health factors include biology, climate, relationships, and schooling.

• A healthy diet, exercise, disease screening, and coping strategies can all improve the health of an individual.

A tool for everyday life, not living intention. Health is a positive concept that emphasizes both social and personal resources and physical capacity. That means health is a tool for promoting the role of a person in a broader society. A healthy lifestyle is a way to live a full life.

More recently, researchers have defined health as a body's ability to adapt to new threats and illnesses. They base this on the idea that, in recent decades, modern science has dramatically increased human awareness of diseases and how they work.

Types

Mental and physical health are the two forms of health most often discussed. They also speak of "spiritual health," "emotional health," and, among others, "financial health." These were also associated with lower levels of stress and mental and physical well-being.

Physical health

Body functions operate at peak performance in a person experiencing physical health due not only to a lack of disease but also to regular exercise, a proper diet, and sufficient rest. When required, we receive treatment to maintain the balance.

Physical wellbeing involves pursuing a healthy lifestyle to reduce disease risk. For example, maintaining physical fitness can protect and improve a person's capacity for breathing and heart function, muscle strength, flexibility, and body composition.

Physical health and wellbeing also help to reduce the risk of an accident or health condition. These include reducing occupational risks, practicing safe sex, maintaining good hygiene, or preventing the use of cigarettes, alcohol, or illicit drugs.

Mental health

Mental health refers to the mental, social, and psychological wellbeing of a person. Mental health is just as important to a true, active lifestyle as physical health.

Defining mental health is more difficult than physical health, as a treatment in many cases relies on the understanding of their experience by the patient. Nevertheless, with advances in testing, certain signs of certain types of mental illness in CT scans and genetic testing are now becoming "seen." Mental health is not just a lack of depression, anxiety, or some other illness. Depends also on the capacity to:

• Enjoy life

- Bounce back from challenging experiences

- To achieve balance

- Adapt to adversity

- Feel safe, and secure

- Reach your potential physical and mental health.

When the chronic disease affects the ability of a person to perform their daily activities, this can contribute, for example, to depression and stress due to money issues. A mental illness such as depression or nervous anorexia may affect the weight and function of the body. It is important that "safety" is viewed as a whole, rather than its different types.

1.2 Associated Factors

If a person wants to live a long and healthy life, there are several positive lifestyle factors that can promote good health. Sure, you can't change your genes or much of the world around you, but making informed and deliberate decisions about diet, exercise, sleep, alcohol use, and smoking can reduce your health risks and potentially add years to your life.

There are huge texts and hundreds of articles you might read about factors that affect your physical well-being with beneficial or negative effects. That said, these six lifestyle changes are the ones that have the best evidence to increase your longevity.

Getting a proper and balance amounts of Sleep

Having a daily and sufficient amount of sleep is first on our list since it is frequently downplayed in terms of diet and exercise value. Several studies have demonstrated the association between sleep and life expectancy, but what scares some people is that the relationship is a U-shaped curve. To put it another way, too little and too much sleep increases mortality (the risk of death).

A good night's sleep is important, no matter what sex or age it may be. Sleep provides an opportunity for your body to recover and regenerate. It not only recharges the proverbial "batteries," but it also performs all the metabolic functions that the body requires, such as regenerating old cells, disposing of waste, and Repairing damage to the cell. For those who give up on the sleep needed to study, remember that sleep is important in memory making, and sleep deprivation leads to forgetfulness.

Even if it's your goal to sleep well, sometimes medical conditions may get in the way. Sleep apnea is a disease that can greatly increase the risks to safety. While the condition affects millions of people, it is thought to be under-diagnosed in large measure. Part of the reason is that there are not always symptoms such as snoring and waking up gasping for air, and sleep apnea can show a variety of unexpected signs and symptoms. It is important to have a word with your doctor about a sleep study if you have any questions as medications (such as CPAP and other interventions) will reduce your risk and improve your life. Changes in your sleep patterns can also be a sign of a change in your health, so if anything changes, see your doctor for a checkup.

Having regular Well-Balanced Meals

A healthy and balanced diet can readily provide energy and reduce the vulnerability to leading chronic diseases such as heart disease, hypertension, diabetes, and cancer. It can also help you keep your weight to normal. Some diseases or conditions have proven ties with specific nutritional or dietary elements.

However, rather than jumping on the latest fad diet, a positive change in dietary lifestyle is what gives maximum protection. Michael Pollan, the founder of eating healthy for life, summed up his advice by saying, "Eat food.

Not too much. Just plants." And of those greens, you have the best chance to get the phytonutrients you need by consuming a rainbow of colors.

Nevertheless, getting some input on what to eat every day is helpful, and this underlies many of the common diet fads. If you're wondering where to start, the Mediterranean diet is abundant in many of the' healthiest' foods and excludes many of the less healthy options.

The more you follow the Mediterranean diet, the lower the risk of developing a host of illnesses. The idea that this dietary strategy is effective is supported by recent studies that looked at more than millions of people and the incidence of more than a dozen chronic diseases. Researchers found that adopting a Mediterranean diet, the risk of health conditions, including heart disease, strokes, cancer, and neurogenerative diseases, was inversely proportional.

Some of the Mediterranean diet's components include fruit and vegetables (a lot), nuts and seeds, fish, whole grains, a strong extra virgin olive oil, and plenty of herbs and spices. Highly processed foods, refined grains, refined oils, and added sugar are not included in the products.

Engaging in Physical Activities on regular basis

Approximately at least thirty minutes a day of regular physical activity adds to health by lowering heart rate, decreasing the risk of cardiovascular disease, and reducing the amount of age-related bone loss and osteoporosis. At this time, it is believed that lack of exercise leads to 9 percent of breast cancers and 10 percent of colon cancers in Europe.

A recent study in Lancet showed that engaging in moderate day-to-day recreational and non-recreational physical activity was associated with a decreased risk of heart disease and total income-free mortality.

Best of all, physical activity can not only be a low-cost way to improve your health (and perhaps your lifespan), but it can even save your money. Think: wash your windows, mow a lawn, sweep a sidewalk, and more. (It is important to note that this level of activity should not be done by those with certain medical conditions.) Once you are 65 years of age, the criteria do not go down, and you may gain from including exercises for strength and flexibility.

You may wonder what researchers mean by exercising at moderate intensity. There are many choices, but it is important to find things that you enjoy and continue to do, such as:

• Gardening

• Walking briskly

• Ballroom dancing

• Bicycling gradually on level ground

• Bathing in the recreation area

Maintaining a balanced healthy Body Weight

Obesity is linked to a shorter lifespan as well as an increased risk of many chronic diseases. The good news is that just being a bit overweight doesn't affect your lifespan, and for those over the age of 65, it's actually better to be on the high side of the average than on the low side.

A research in 2018 (part of the Framingham heart report) analyzed body mass index and mortality over a 24-year period. (Normal body mass index ranges from 19 to 24.) For those who were obese, those with a body mass index of 30 to 35 had a 27% rise in mortality, and those with a body mass index of 35 to 40 had a 93% increase.

What's the ideal weight?

Mortality had been increased among those who also smoked among those who were overweight but not obese (had a body mass index between 25 and 30). People with a high-level body mass had the lowest mortality rate.

There is no true magic when it comes to maintaining (or attaining) a typical level of body mass. The real "secret" is eating a healthy diet (not too much and avoiding empty calories) and exercising on a daily basis (even if it's fun things like gardening).

Eating breakfast has been emphasized as required for optimum health in the past. Science is changing the thinking now, and extended fasting (without feeding for 13 hours or more every day) may have some advantages. Although the idea and evidence to support it are new, intermittent fasting can help with weight loss and also seem to have benefits in reducing cancer risk. Talk to your doctor if you're struggling. However, keep in mind that fad diets don't work, and the best chance of success is to follow healthy eating habits over the long term and participate in regular physical activity for life.

Avoid Using Tobacco Products

Smoking alone in the world accounts for so many deaths a year. Adding to this are millions of people living while struggling with a smoking-related illness. If you want to live an enjoyable life, don't smoke or chew tobacco for as long as you live.

The list of smoking-related diseases and cancers is lengthy, but sometimes long-range concerns quickly change less than immediate concerns.

If you're struggling to leave, worrying about immediate consequences will help. Maybe the cost or social nature of being a smoker was banned in many cases while smoking.

Or maybe the effects of the mid-range would inspire you. Smoking speeds up wrinkling for women (and men).

In people, it's not just the arteries that supply the tobacco-affected heart. Smaller arteries are damaged similarly in another region of the body, and a significant association exists between smoking and erectile dysfunction.

Drinking alcohol in moderation or not at All

Even with the hype over red wine and longevity, alcohol should only be consumed in moderation, and not at all for many people. Red wine (in moderation) has been found to offer protection from diseases ranging from heart disease to Alzheimer's disease, but to get these benefits, you don't need to drink red wine.

Red wine is rich in flavonoids, especially the resveratrol of the phytonutrients. Nevertheless, resveratrol is also present in red grape juice, red grapes, and peanuts too.

A moderate consumption (one drink for women, two for men) can decrease heart disease. Still, the correlation between alcohol and breast cancer indicates that caution should be exercised even with this level. People who have three drinks a week have a 15 percent higher risk of breast cancer, and the chance for each extra drink they have each day goes up by another 10 percent.

Higher alcohol levels can cause health and behavioral problems, including an increased risk of high blood pressure, stroke, and heart disease, certain cancers, injuries, crime, suicide, and deaths in general.

To celebrate a particular moment, and when achieved in moderation after all, mental and social wellbeing rank right up there with a modest intake of alcohol in physical health, by those who have no alcohol problem and are not predisposed to alcohol abuse, maybe part of a healthy lifestyle. So long as everyone present is well aware of the dangers of alcohol before drinking to your toast.

These six lifestyle habits can go a long way in improving the chances of a long, healthy life you'll lead. Yet we know life goes beyond good health, and equally important is mental, social, and spiritual wellbeing. Exercising stress management, cultivating a passion or hobby, and sometimes pampering yourself should be high on your to-do list.

Yet even when people do everything right, physical illness or mental stress cannot always be avoided. Many health professionals now believe that "rolling with the punches" of life, or exhibiting resilience, is a skill that we should all cultivate if we wish to live our best life today.

Factors for good health

Good health is affected by a wide range of factors. A person is born with a variety of genes, and in some people an uncommon genetic pattern can lead to a level of health that is less than optimum. Environmental factors play an important role. The environment alone sometimes suffices for health impacts. Many times an environmental stimulus in a genetically susceptible individual will cause illness.

Access to health care plays a role, but the WHO indicates that the following factors could have a greater impact on health than this:

- Where a person lives

- Condition of the climate

- The biology

- Employment

- Level of education

- Relationships with friends and family

The economic and social climate that involves how wealthy a family or society is.

The physical environment which includes parasites present in an area, or levels of pollution. Characteristics and habits of the individual which Include the genes with which a person is born and their lifestyle choices. According to the WHO, the higher the socioeconomic status of a person, the greater the probability of enjoying good health, good education, a well-paid job, affording good health care when threatened with health.

People having lower end socioeconomic status are more likely to experience pressures related to their daily lives, such as financial difficulties, marital instability, and unemployment, as well as social factors such as marginalization and prejudice. All of these lead to poor health risks.

A low socioeconomic status also means less healthcare access. People in developed countries with universal healthcare systems have longer life expectancies than those without universal healthcare in developed countries.

Cultural problems can have an impact on health. A society's practices and customs and the reaction of a family to them can have a good or bad health impact. For example, people around the Mediterranean are more likely to eat high levels of fruit, vegetables, and olive, and eat as a family, compared to cultures with high fast-food consumption.

How does a person handle stress affect his or her health? People who smoke, drink, or take drugs to forget their problems are likely to have more health problems later than someone who has a healthy diet and exercise to combat stress.

Men and women are susceptible to various factors relating to health. Women may be at greater risk of poor health in societies where women earn less than men or are less educated than men.

Preserving health

The best way to maintain wellness is to protect it through a healthy lifestyle, rather than waiting for things to get better until we're sick. This state of enhanced wellbeing is called wellbeing.

According to the McKinley Health Center wellness as it is a state of optimal wellbeing that is geared towards maximizing the potential of an individual. It is a life-long process of moving towards improving your physical, intellectual, emotional, social, spiritual, and environmental wellbeing.

Wellness encourages positive awareness and engagement in wellness, as an adult and as a society. It is a lifelong, daily dedication to preserving the longevity and good health.

Steps that can help us to maximize our health include:

• A balanced, nutritious diet, obtained as naturally as possible

• Regular exercise

• Disease screening that may present a risk

• Learning how to tackle stress

• Extensively engaging in activities that provide purpose and connection with others

• Maintaining a positive outlook and appreciating what you have

• Defining a value system and putting it into action.

For each individual, peak health will be different, and how you achieve wellness can be different from the way someone else does it. It may not be possible to prevent illness completely, but doing our best to improve resilience and prepare the body and mind to cope with problems as they arise is a measure that we can all take.

1.2 What Difference does it makes?

What might it do well for someone? One wants to think his / her body is like a race car. When they put in low-grade petrol, the result will be worse. Healthy eating helps with muscle cramping is often felt. It just feels so much better and more vigorous too.

This doesn't mean you shouldn't eat burgers or something you like. The theory is that these types of food should be consumed in moderation. Before a big performance or workout, you would be hard-pressed to find athletes of any quality eating greasy, nutrient-poor foods.

A healthy lifestyle has health benefits in both the short and the long term. Long-term eating a balanced diet, regular exercise, and keeping a healthy weight can add years to your life and reduce the risk of certain diseases, including cancer, diabetes, cardiovascular disease, osteoporosis, and obesity. The sole basis of being healthy is not physical fitness; being healthy means being mentally and emotionally fit. Keeping safe should be an integral part of your lifestyle. Living a healthy lifestyle can help prevent long-term illnesses and chronic diseases. It's critical for your self-esteem and self-image to feel good about yourself and take care of your health. Keep a healthy lifestyle by doing what's best for your body. If you want to be a healthy and well-rounded person, here are a few staying safe tips that can help you do just that:

1. Maintain a regular exercise routine

Keep that in mind, at the gym, you don't have to push yourself into intense workouts, but you must stay as healthy as you can. You should stick to simple exercises on the floor, swim, walk, or simply keep going by doing some household chores. Do what your body's makes you do?

What's crucial is you keep on exercising.

Give a workout of at least twenty to thirty minutes a day at least three to five days a week. Have a routine; ensure you get enough physical activity every day.

2. Be extra conscious in your diet

You need to keep eating well, to maintain a healthy lifestyle. Add more fruits and vegetables and eat fewer sugar, high sodium and saturated fat in your diet. Avoid eating candy and junk food.

Stop skipping a meal; this will only make the moment you start eating more food your body craves. Remember burning up more calories than eating.

3. Engage in the stuff you are passionate about

To keep up the stress and life demands from taking over, take a break every now and then to do something you love to do.

You must surround yourself with positive energy to have a stable mental and emotional state. Sure, you can't avoid all of the issues. Yet, with an optimistic outlook, it helps overcome these obstacles. Surround yourself with supportive friends and people who will each time give you constructive criticism to help you improve.

Make it a habit of always looking at life's brighter side. If you think you find yourself in the worst situation, something good and positive is always an upside to it. Instead, focus on those issues.

It's not that difficult to maintain a healthy lifestyle, nor does it require a lot of effort. Only keep doing what you do and apply the aforementioned staying safe tips — sure you'll be a well-rounded individual in no time.

The impact of good health

Do you know healthy habits like eating well, exercising, and avoiding harmful substances are important, but have you ever stopped thinking about why you follow them? Any behavior that supports your physical, mental, and emotional health is a healthy habit. Such habits make you feel good and improve your overall health.

This is obvious that healthy habits are difficult to develop, and often require a change of attitude. But if you're willing to sacrifice to improve your health, it can have a far-reaching effect regardless of your age, sex, or physical ability. Here are five healthy lifestyle benefits.

Controls weight

Eating well and daily workouts will help you avoid overweight gain and maintain a healthy weight. It's essential to be physically active to achieve your weight-loss goals. Even if you don't try to lose weight, regular exercise will enhance cardiovascular health, strengthen your immune system, and increase your level of energy.

For each week, plan for a minimum of 150 minutes of moderate physical activity. When you can't spend this amount of time exercising, look for easy ways to increase exercise all day. Try walking instead of driving, for example, taking the stairs instead of the elevator, or speed while talking on the phone.

This can also help control weight by eating a healthy, calorie-managed diet. You stop being too hungry later when you start the day with a healthy breakfast, which could send you running to get fast food before lunch.

Skipping breakfast can also raise your blood sugar, which increases fat storage. Incorporate at least five portions of fruit and vegetables into your daily diet. Such foods, low in calories and high in nutrients, are helping to regulate weight. Restrict sugary beverage intakes, such as soft drinks and fruit juices, and pick lean meats such as tuna and turkey.

Improves mood

Having done well for your body always pays off for your mind. Physical activity increases endorphin development. Endorphins are chemicals in the brain, which make you feel happier and more relaxed. Eating a healthy diet and exercising can lead to the improved physique. You'll feel better about your looks, which can improve your self-esteem and confidence. Short-term exercise effects include reducing stress and increasing cognitive function.

It's not only diet and exercise that lead to mood improvement. Another healthy habit which leads to improved mental health is social connections. Whether it's volunteering, joining a club, or watching a film, social activities help to improve morale and mental functioning by regulating the levels of the mind active and serotonin. Don't get in isolation. Spend time in regular intervals with family or friends, if not every day. When physical distance occurs between you and your loved ones, use the technology to stay connected. Pick up your phone or launch a chat video.

Combats diseases

Healthy habits help to avoid such complications of health, such as heart disease, stroke, and high blood pressure. You will keep your cholesterol and blood pressure within a safe range if you take care of yourself. That keeps your blood flowing smoothly, reducing your cardiovascular disease risk.

Regular physical activity and a proper diet can also avoid or help you deal with a wide range of health issues, including:

- Metabolic syndrome

- Diabetes

- Depression

- Other types of cancer

- Arthritis

Make sure that you schedule a physical examination regularly. The doctor will monitor the weight, pulse, and blood pressure and will take a sample of your urine and blood. The appointment will show a great deal about your wellbeing. Follow-up with your doctor is crucial, and listen to any advice to improve your health.

Boosts energy

Since eating too much unsanitary food, we all felt a lethargic feeling. Whenever you eat a balanced diet, your body gets the fuel; it needs to manage your level of energy. A healthy diet includes:

• Whole grains

• Lean meats

• Low-fat dairy products

• Fruits

• Vegetables

Regular physical activity often strengthens muscle strength and increases endurance, giving you more energy. Exercise helps supply your tissues with oxygen and nutrients, which lets your cardiovascular system work more efficiently so that you have enough energy to carry out your daily activities. It also encourages better sleep by helping to improve capacity. It allows you to sleep quicker and to sleep deeper.

Lack of sleep can cause a range of problems. Beyond feeling tired and sluggish, if you don't get enough sleep, you can feel irritable and moody too.

What's more, poor quality of sleep may be responsible for high blood pressure, diabetes, and heart disease, and may shorten the life expectancy as well.

To improve the quality of the sleep, stick to a routine where you wake up and go to bed every night at the same time. Reduce the intake of caffeine, limit the napping, and create a comfortable environment for sleep. Turn off the lights and the TV, and keep the room temperature high.

Improves longevity

By practicing healthy habits, you are boosting your chances of a longer life. An eight-year study of 13,000 people, reported by the American Council on Exercise. The study showed that those who walked for only 30 minutes each day significantly reduced their risk of premature death relative to those who never exercised. Looking forward to spending more time with your loved ones is justification enough to start walking. Start with quick5-minute walks and increase the time slowly until you are up to 30 minutes away.

Poor habits are hard to break, so you won't regret this decision until you follow a healthier lifestyle. Healthy habits reduce the risk of certain illnesses, improve your physical appearance and mental health, and provide a much-needed boost to your energy level. You're not going to change your attitude and actions immediately, so be careful and one day at a time.

Chapter 2: Root Causes of weak Health

Poor health study will be debated in relation to the life cycle and society. The emphasis on root causes that are closely linked to poor health standards will be highlighted in the circumstances under which people are born, develop, live, function, and age (shaped by the distribution of wealth, power, and resources at global, regional, and local levels). They are also described as' factors that contribute to the current state of health of an individual that can be of a biological, financial, psychosocial, behavioral, or social nature.

2.1 Life Cycle

In order to explore the effect of a life cycle on health awareness and incentives for healthy behavior, most people, especially for children in developing countries, health outcomes, are largely determined by decisions taken within the household, in particular by the family and the mother and father. Parents provide (or fail to provide) everything from nutrition and shelter to education and health care, from infancy to adulthood. Additionally, the family is usually the center of care and support for the disabled, who, in turn, also contribute to childcare. Models are designed to position public health policies and programs within the family and external forces that affect the actions of a family.

Such models of the lifecycle, which we term the "family health cycle," link infants, mothers, fathers, and grandparents in a framework that forms the health of individual family members as a whole.

In addition, the family or household communicates with various community participants, the formal and informal health services network, and is influenced by a wide array of external conditions and inputs. Generally, the matter starts with the birth of a child, who, as an infant boy or girl, passes through the first stage of the process, becomes a teenager, and enters adolescence. At this point, the individual is biologically "free" to go through another stage of the cycle as a parent, and then as a grandparent, barring early adult mortality or offspring, childlessness can go through the mechanism once again. Each stage carries health risks unique to age and gender, and thus calls for various health interventions. Interventions at each stage can be seen as inputs to help individuals survive (and benefit from lower morbidity) until the next stage requires new inputs for intervention. Such an idea and framework helps identify what types of biomedical, social, economic, and environmental interventions are likely to be most effective at each stage of the cycle. It thus has the potential to enhance understanding of the linkages among the many available interventions and to help make better use of scarce public health resources.

Nutrition through the lifecycle

The nutritional and energy-change needs of an individual over the life span. For example, while a typical adult woman may need only 6.7 mg of calcium per pound of body weight, a nine-month-old child requires 27 mg of calcium per pound of body weight.

The need for nutrients is highest during rising periods of a body, which arise in childhood, in puberty, and during pregnancy. Once the period of growth has stopped, energy needs and the need for certain nutrients decreases.

The reasons behind a person's food choices often differ over the life span as social, psychological, cultural, and leisure roles shift over that period of time.

For starters, peer views and perceptions about body image become particularly important during the teenage years. By comparison, adults are more likely to be affected by their health needs.

Infants

The member's manual addresses strategies for breastfeeding and bottle-feeding. Research shows breastfeeding is healthy for both mom and baby. When teens know about the benefits of breastfeeding, when they're parents, they may be more likely to consider it.

Generations ago, the preferred method of feeding was breastfeeding. Bottle feeding became more popular as formulation became readily available. At the same time, a movement towards feeding solid food to babies at an early age also became common. Today, baby feeding patterns are changing once more. Breastfeeding has gained in popularity due to the nutritional benefits and antibodies that breast milk offers for the baby (to protect against infection and allergies).

Early Childhood

Young kids like to feed themselves just like they like to do all the things for themselves. Spilling the milk and making other messes is simple when they know how to eat! In providing:

• Tiny utensils that are easy to hold, parents and babysitters can help young kids learn to eat and feed themselves.

• Edged plates to avoid food from falling off the platter.

• Small cups that are not going to tip easily over.

• Foods that you can pick and eat with your fingers.

• Because too much can be daunting, small portions of food on a plate.

• High chair, booster seat, or table cushions.

Kids who feel optimistic at family meals are more likely to develop healthier attitudes. This is an opportunity to improve good eating habits and to add a wide variety of foods. Food should nevertheless, not be used to relax or encourage children. That can lead to children associating desires with food and not hunger.

Kids have tiny stomachs and, at one point, cannot consume much food. Eating many snacks and treats is better than eating three large meals a day. Bite-sized pieces of raw fruit and vegetables, as well as cheese cubes, are perfect snacks. The following include other delicious, nutritious snacks.

Overall, health does not rely on a single meal or diet but on making good dietary decisions over time. There are typically nutritious substitutes that can be supplemented by the foods which a child refuses to eat. The following tips could help to make food fun.

• Use the cookie cutters to make animals or toy made sandwiches.

• Make ribbons, pinwheels (curled-up sandwich), or anything else.

Shape foods like turkey, ham, or low-fat bologna roll-ups in unusual ways. For older children, toothpicks in the shapes of boats or buildings can hold the cut vegetables.

• Paint faces on peeled fruits, such as bananas, oranges, or tangerines. Or split a fruit in half, like a peach, spread with yogurt or low-fat cream cheese, and add raisins or other dried fruit pieces to a fruit nose.

• Make a sandwich facial. The "glue" maybe peanut butter. To the eyes, seek raisins. Try jerseys for eyelashes and eyebrows. Consider Carrot curls for yellow hair. Give a tip on a carrot for a nose. Consider a slice of red pepper for a mouthful. Add carrot or celery sticks to the arms and feet.

Television is another factor that contributes to food selection. The foods advertised on television affect children. Before the age of seven or eight, few children may think critically of those advertised foods and may beg parents to buy a frequently advertised food.

Some kids don't like milk or some dairy products. There are nutritional alternatives to "sneak" milk in a child's diet, although some parents may be very concerned.

Include other foods and mixtures that include milk and/or other dairy products such as:

- Pie,

- Pasta,

- Creamy soups,

- Macaroni and cheese,

- Tacos or meat burritos.

What's up with ice cream? Ice cream, ice tea, and frozen yogurt are made of milk in order to find calcium and other nutrients in milk. They're still higher in fat and sugar, though. Occasionally, ice cream can be counted as a serving from the food group Dairy, Yogurt, and Cheese, but when this occurs, the use of other fats and sweets should be removed.

If a child has trouble digesting milk, some options include:

- One-time drinking of a small amount,

- Consuming yogurt or cheese,

- Consumption milk added to lactase. Lactase is an enzyme that breaks down the sugar (lactose) in milk. Lactase tablets can be attached to your own.

Teenage Years

A child's body starts a period of rapid size change and develops at ten years of age in girls and 12 years in boys.

This is called the "adolescent growth spurt." An average girl can grow 10 inches taller over the next four years and gain between 40 and 50 pounds. An average boy can grow taller by 12 inches and earn between 50 and 60 pounds. The body shape also begins to change at the same time.

The spurt of teenage development requires a great many different nutrients. Calcium is particularly important for bone growth and health because, during puberty, 45 percent of the bone that an adult has is formed.

Although some teenagers are worried that they don't develop as quickly as their school friends or other classmates, there is wide variation in the age at which the spurts of adolescent development begin. This usually depends more on the genetic characteristics than on being a certain age.

How a person feels about his body is closely linked to how they feel about themselves. It's crucial for adolescents to:

• Know that change is natural,

• Take care of their bodies, and

• Speak to family members and friends who endorse it.

It is important to emphasize that changes in body size and shape are part of normal adolescent development. Females gain proportionally more body fat during this time, while males gain proportionally more muscle and bone mass.

One of the changes taking place during adolescence is the varying hormonal levels in the body. These hormones are responsible for the changes seen in the physical development of the body and secondary characteristics such as facial hair growth and deepening voices.

It's important to stress that changes in body size and shape are part of the normal development of teenagers.

During this time, females gain proportionally more body fat, while males gain proportionally more muscle and bone mass. One of the changes occurring during adolescence is the varying hormonal levels in the organism. Such hormones are responsible for the changes seen in the body's physical development and secondary features such as facial hair growth and voice deepening.

Pregnancy

Pregnancy is a special time within the life of a woman. Healthy eating can increase the possibility of having a healthy baby. Gradual weight gain is important; 2-4 pounds for the first three months, then just under 1 pound per week for the rest of the pregnancy. It is advised to get a total gain of 25-35 pounds.

If at the beginning of the pregnancy, a woman is overweight, she should not diet, but rather limit the number of desserts and other "extras." She needs to continue a steady weight gain line.

If a woman is underweight at the start of pregnancy, she will increase her intake of food and follow a steady line of weight gain.

In addition, a pregnant woman has different water and fluid requirements, including:

• Drink at least 6-8 cups of fluid daily;

• Limit the amount of caffeine-containing beverages;

• Limit soft drinks and sugary drinks; and

• Consume moderately aspartame-containing and saccharin-containing drinks.

All the weight gained goes directly to tissue stores for the baby and the mother. Since the baby receives most weight gain, a small weight gain may mean a baby too small.

Lifestyle and poor nutritional habits of a pregnant woman can lead to a baby with low birth weight (less than 5 1/2 pounds). Babies with less birth weight are more likable to:

• Breathing deficiency due to poor production of the lungs;

• Brain damage due to insufficient nutrition;

• Anemia (less red blood cells) due to insufficient nutrition or lack of time to store the iron needed;

• Low body temperatures due to lack of fat stored to keep warm; and

• Bleeding in the brain. It happens to 40-45 percent of babies born too small; it leads to brain damage or death.

Babies with low birth weight are associated with 70 percent of infant deaths. In particular, low birthweight babies are associated with the following habits:

• Poor nutrition,

• Smoking cigarettes,

• Drinking alcohol,

• Opioid use and

• Lack of early and frequent prenatal medical checkups.

Older Adults

Three of the keys to good health throughout a lifetime have been: • eat a variety of nutritious foods;

• Limit the amount of fat, salt and sugar in the diet, and

• Regular exercise.

While these keys can't guarantee good health, they can help a person stay healthy as they grow older or maybe improve health. Older adults, however, often have specific nutritional needs because:

• To remain at the same weight, they need fewer calories than younger ones; and

• Other health problems become more common as people grow older.

The need for calories decreases around 5 percent every ten years after the teen years. A 60-year-old therefore requires 20 percent fewer calories than the same weight of a 20-year-old. The best way to stay at the same weight for older adults is to:

• Eat less, and/or

• Work out more.

The vitamin and mineral needs of stable older adults seem close to those of younger adults, although few studies have been performed on the elderly's nutritional requirements. Recent studies have shown that while older adults need fewer calories, protein and calcium needs have been somewhat higher in older adults relative to younger ones. One theory might be that older adults consume those nutrients less quickly. In this way, older adults should be encouraged to consume recommended amounts of protein foods like milk, particularly because of their refusal of meat and milk is a common problem among older adults. Excess protein should be avoided, however, as with other age groups.

Many older adults struggle to chew and swallow food. Resolving these issues is vital to elderly people's nutritional status. The following suggestions for easy chewing and swallowing protein-rich foods may be helpful:

• Vegetables served in a cream or cheese sauce;

• Raw fruits and vegetables chopped or rubbed in a gelatin salad;

• Eggs cooked in any way;

• Legumes, such as split peas, navy beans, lima beans, pinto beans, and kidney beans;

• Fish; and

• Ground meats or finely chopped meats.

Another hallmark concern for the elderly is decreased thirst. Although the urine is normally collected in the kidney to preserve body water, the elderly appear to excrete diluted urine. The aging kidney also loses its working units and is less able to cope with pain. This condition will lead to a decrease in the amount of body fluids; the composition of these body fluids can also alter, which can potentially be fatal.

Making sure older people drink enough water to offset fluid losses is extremely important. A serious threat to the elderly is dehydration. Fruit juices, milk, and even coffee, tea, soft drinks, "ades," ice creams, and gelatin desserts are mostly sugar. Fluids at mealtimes should not be allowed to replace food but should be provided at meals and encouraged between meals.

Eight Signs of Poor Nutrition

The right amounts of food are key to a long and healthy life, and the needs of your body change as you age. You don't need as many calories, for example, but you need more of a few nutrients like vitamin D and calcium. And as you age, the body may have trouble taking vitamins found in foods such as B12 and using them there.

Because of this, older adults do not always get the necessary nutrients. Knowing the signs of poor nutrition can be a good idea, so if you notice any of them, you can talk with your doctor.

1. Feeling Tired

If you're always losing strength, it can be a sign that you're not getting enough of some nutrients, including iron. If there is a deficiency and you don't have enough red blood cells to transport oxygen and nutrients into parts of your body, too little of that mineral will contribute to anemia.

Fatigue can also be a symptom of certain health conditions, such as cardiac disease or a thyroid problem.

2. Brittle, Dry Hair

Nutrients such as iron, folate, and vitamin C are essential to your hair. You might notice some unhealthy changes in it if you don't get enough of these through your diet. Your skin could be thin and pale too.

But other health conditions, like a thyroid problem, can also affect the hair and skin.

3. Ridged or Spoon-Shaped Nails

Poor nutrition can cause multiple changes to the nails. Like your hair, the nails may become thin and brittle, but there may also be other signs. One is the nails curving like a spoon, especially on your index finger or third finger. That could mean that you're low on fuel.

The nails may also be ridged or start falling apart from the surface of the nail. In addition to problems with iron, low levels of protein, calcium, or vitamins A, B6, C, and D may cause nail problems.

4. Dental Problems

Your mouth is one of the first locations where it can show signs of poor nutrition. A lack of vitamin C will cause gingivitis (gum disease) to bleed, irritate gums. You might even lose your teeth in severe cases.

If you have dentures or missing or loose teeth, your food choices will alter. Poor nutrition then turns into a double-edged sword: If your mouth hurts and you have trouble with your teeth, eating healthy foods is even more challenging. And this makes keeping your teeth cleaner.

5. Change in Bowel Habits

Constipation can happen if you don't get enough fiber, found in whole grains, fruits, and vegetables.

6. Mood and Mental Health Issues

For depression, an unhealthy diet may play a part. It can influence various mental activities and cause you to lose interest in things you used to enjoy. You may also feel disoriented and lose your memory.

7. Easy Bruising and Slow Healing

If you bruise easily, particularly if there is no obvious reason for this (such as falling down or bumping into something), your diet can play a part. Specifically, you can lack protein, vitamin C, or vitamin K, both required to heal wounds. Vitamin C helps repair tissue itself, and vitamin K is essential for blood coagulation.

8. Slow Immune Response

Without proper nutrition, your immune system may not be as strong as it needs to be in combating illness. Protein and zinc are among the most important nutrients for a strong immune system, along with vitamins A, C, and E.

How to Stay Healthy

A balanced diet of fruits, vegetables, lean proteins, whole grains, low-fat dairy, and healthier oils are the best way to prevent these kinds of problems. At each meal, choose a range of these foods to get the vitamins and minerals you need. And seek to limit packaged or processed foods and baked goods high in saturated and trans fats.

2.2 Social determinants of health

Quite often the very first thing that comes to mind when we talk about wellness is physicians or clinics, or perhaps the choices we make about our diet, or whether we exercise, smoke, or drink alcohol.

Yet did you know that the critical ingredients for a healthy life for most people are, in fact, a right home, a good education, a decent job, friendships and networks to feel part of?

These are often called "private" or "greater" health determinants. For more information on the root causes of ill health and the things that make us happy read this A-Z.

A - Avoidable inequalities

Some classes of people in our society seem to have better health than others. While the amount of money/income, we have can decide how safe we are, we also see health disparities related to a learning disability, gender, race, age, orientation, or religion. These are "health disparities" but should not be seen as unavoidable in fact; they are both preventable and unjust.

B - Behaviors

Thinking about staying healthy for many people means contemplating our behaviors; in other words, the choices we take while buying food or whether we are exercising, smoking, or drinking alcohol. Nevertheless, the evidence is clear that while factors such as these habits, our genetic make-up, and access to health care play a role in how healthy we are, the conditions in which we are born, live, and work have a more significant impact.

C - Causes of illness

One way to understand what makes us alive is to find the "causes of the causes."

The Health Foundation states in their useful guide' What makes us healthy': "What causes heart disease, for example? Arteries Blocked? But what does block those arteries?

It could be food which is unhealthy, lack of exercise or stress. But what shapes our choices for food and drink, and our opportunities to be involved, or makes us feel stressed? The answers lie in the circumstances we are born, we live, and we work in."

D - Diet

Maintaining a proper diet is an effective way to stay healthy, but not everyone has the same nutritious food exposure. For example, there is a higher density of fast food outlets in more deprived areas and less access to healthy food. Our food environment shapes our choices.

E-Education

Having a good education helps us get a decent job, and our ability to make informed decisions increases. In contrast, poor literacy is linked to poorer health and prospects for future employment.

F - Financial resources

It can be easier to avoid stress if your family has a healthy income, make healthier choices, and feel like you have a financial safety net if things go wrong.

G - Gap

To show the effects of inequality, health experts frequently talk of the "difference" in life expectancy between the worlds' most and least deprived areas. Men in richest areas live 9.4 years longer than men in the poorest regions. Among females, this same gap is 7.4 years.

H - Housing

Having a safe and appropriate home in which to live helps us stay healthy while hot, cold, or overcrowded accommodation raises our risk of asthma, COPD, trips and drops, and poor mental health.

I - Impact on the economy

Trying to make our society safer and fairer is socially the right thing to do, but it is also economically so. For example, in larger hospitalizations alone, the additional cost of health inequality is about billions of dollars a year. Health disparities are also impacting jobs and growth, which cost our national and local economies.

J - Jobs

There is definitely a clear evidence that having a job improves our overall health and wellbeing. Beyond providing us with money, having a good job gives us meaning and security, keeps us busy, and gives us a social network.

K - Knowledge

Limited health knowledge (often referred to as "health literacy") is linked to unhealthy behaviors such as poor diet, smoking, and lack of physical activity. It is associated with an increased risk of disease and death.

People with limited health literacy are less likely to use preventive services. They are more likely to use emergency services, are less likely to manage long-term health conditions successfully, resulting in higher costs for health care. The health literacy of a person tends to be related to his or her social situation.

L - Localities/places

Since our environments–how we are raised, live, and work–are so closely linked to how happy we are, local places and societies play a significant role in keeping us alive.

Local authorities and voluntary sector organizations should work together to reduce health disparities, both through the conventional services they provide and through enhancing community life, building social connections, and giving public people a voice in local decisions.

M - Meaning and purpose

People who live healthier and happier lives are linked to their families, friends, and local networks. As being an active part of a community, whether it be through work, clubs, or social activities, gives our lives a sense of purpose that enhances our wellbeing.

N - healthcare

Health care is often only one of many factors that affect how safe we are when we talk about our health.

We have different national health systems, so how can it be that some countries have better health rates while others have poorer health? It suggests that ill health is more closely linked to our climate–such as poverty levels–than it is to healthcare.

O - Outdoor spaces

Well-designed outdoor spaces improve the health and safety of those who regularly use them, reduce the risk of falling, encourage physical activity, and reduce social isolation. Even in urban areas, we can enhance our physical and mental health by having access to the natural environment, such as parks, gardens, woods, or waterways. There is enough information on how local areas can use their planning system to build safe places.

P - Pollution

Air pollution is the biggest environmental danger to health and there is good evidence that it has a significant impact on the incidence and frequency of cardiovascular disease and lung health, among other things. It has both short-and long-term effects on health and has a particular impact on children as they develop.

Often the most socioeconomically vulnerable suffer the most

from pollution's health effects.

Certain disproportionately affected groups include the elderly, infants, pregnant women and individuals with existing medical conditions.

Q - Quality of life

Health is not only about the length of life we live, but also about our quality of life and there is a massive gap between the wealthiest and most impoverished regions. The difference between the first world's most and least deprived areas in healthy life expectancy (years spent in good health) is around 19 years. In other words, people living in the most deprived regions spend about a third of their lives in poor health, compared to just about a sixth for people living in the least deprived areas.

R - Resilience

Human resilience is correlated with attitudes, thoughts, and actions, encouraging personal wellbeing and mental health. Strengthening and building resilience is, therefore, critical and can be accomplished by learning better skills and strategies to manage stress and better ways of thinking about the challenges of life with support from the family, friends, neighbors, and faith communities.

S - Social isolation

Connecting with other people counts. Research shows that our mental and physical health is severely deprived of social connections. Anyone may feel social isolation and loneliness, but this is considered more generally in later life.

When our population ages, the number of older people is growing, and we are seeing an increase in the number of people with chronic and extreme loneliness. Yes, older people will go a whole month without talking to a friend, neighbor, or family member.

T - Transport

Many deprived areas tend to have a higher central road density resulting in lower air quality, higher noise levels, and higher traffic crash rates. One approach is to encourage active travel. Switching to walking or cycling all or a part of our journeys can improve health, quality of life, and the environment. There is ample information on how local areas can use their planning system to design good places.

U - Unemployment

Being unemployed can undermine our health and increase our risk of long-term illness, including poor mental health and cardiovascular disease.

V - Vulnerable people

Some of the most extreme health inequalities affect the most vulnerable in society, such as people who are homeless, prisoners, migrants, drug users, and sex workers.

W - Wider determinants

Health experts also speak about the "larger health determinants" This term refers to the variety of social, economic, and environmental factors that influence the mental and physical health of individuals.

Y - Years of life lost

Known disease-related risks are similar in both rich and poor areas (smoking, unhealthy diet, alcohol consumption, etc.). But the years of being wasted in more deprived areas due to these habits are often as much as double those in wealthy neighborhoods.

Z - Zero to two - having a good start in life

A child's brain shows a remarkable ability to absorb information and adapt to its environment during the first two years of life.

Therefore, successful early experience is critical to ensuring that children are ready for learning, ready for school, and have good life chances.

Chapter 3: Fuel up with diet

There are different kinds of foods and herbs that affect health differently. Different foods and herbs can be helpful by elevating the eating plans strategically. Eating a healthy diet is not about rigid limits, keeping unrealistically slim, or depriving yourself of the food you enjoy. It's about feeling great, getting more time, enhancing your health, and boosting your mood, instead.

It clearly does not have to be that overly complicated to eat healthily. When you feel overwhelmed by all of the contradictory dietary and health recommendations out there, you're not alone. It seems you'll find another saying the exact opposite for every expert who tells you a particular food is right for you. The truth is that while it has been shown that certain specific foods or nutrients have a beneficial effect on mood, the most important thing is your overall dietary pattern. The foundation of a healthy diet should be to replace processed food whenever possible, with real food. Eating food as close to nature as possible will make a massive difference in the way you think, look, and feel.

The fundamentals of healthy eating

While some extreme diets may say otherwise, to sustain a healthy body, we all need a combination of protein, fat, carbohydrates, nutrients, vitamins, and minerals in our diets. You don't have to exclude all types of food from your diet, but instead choose the healthiest choices in each category.

Protein gives you the ability to get up and go and start while improving mood and cognitive function as well. Consuming too much protein can be harmful to people with kidney disease, but recent research suggests that many of us, particularly as we age, need more high-quality protein.

That really doesn't mean you need to consume more animal products every day from a range of plant-based protein sources that can ensure your body gets all the necessary protein it needs.

Not all fat is equal. While bad fats can ruin your diet and increase the risk of certain diseases, good fats protect your heart and brain. Yes, healthy fats like omega-3s are essential to your wellbeing, both physically and emotionally. Including healthier fat in your diet will help improve your mood, increase your wellbeing, and even change your waistline.

Eating high in dietary fiber foods (grains, fruits, vegetables, nuts, and beans) will help you stay healthy and reduce your risk of heart disease, stroke, and diabetes; It can also make your skin more youthful, and even help you lose weight.

By not consuming enough calcium in your diet can also contribute to anxiety, depression, and sleeping difficulties, as well as leading to osteoporosis. Whatever your age or gender, having calcium-rich foods in your diet, avoiding those that deplete calcium, and getting enough magnesium and vitamins D and K to help calcium do its job is important.

Carbohydrate is one of the primary sources of energy in your body. However, most should come from complex, unrefined carbs (vegetables, whole grains, fruit) instead of sugars and refined carbs. Cutting back on white bread, pastries, starches, and sugar can prevent swift spikes in blood sugar, mood, and energy fluctuations, and fat build-up, especially around your waistline.

3.1 Healthy foods

Buying healthy food doesn't just mean you're going to eat delicious foods; if you're eating healthy foods, you're helping to improve your overall health, whether its muscle-building, sharpening your mind, or strengthening your core.

Make sure your grocery list contains as many of these foods as possible the next time you drop by the market or order food delivery.

Each of the planet's 100 healthiest foods has specific health-promoting powers to contribute to your healthiest and happiest life.

Fruits & Vegetables

Newsflash: Vegetables will help with weight loss! Okay, all right, we're admitting that's not exactly breaking news, but did you know that some veggies reign supreme when it comes to rapid weight loss while others fall relatively flat in comparison? That is true! Thanks to their specific nutritional profiles, some product-aisle picks can help you trim down by reviving your metabolism, turning off the fatty belly genes and frying flab, and that's on top of all the other health-boosting benefits. Read on to find out which delicious picks fit the bill, and find out how to incorporate them into your diet.

Skip your next few months of a fad diet. Put aside specific diets that help you to lose weight. You should instead concentrate on filling the body with healthy food as a way of life. Eating these healthy foods will not only aid in weight loss but will also improve your overall health and well-being. Your approach towards longevity is to add the healthiest meals possible. It's easy to ask which food is healthiest.

A vast number of foods are nutritious, as well as savory. Through filling your plate with fruits, vegetables, high-quality protein, and other whole grains, you will have colorful, nutritious, and healthy meals for you.

All too often, apparently healthy snacks are loaded secretly with sugar, saturated fats, and carbohydrates.

That's why we picked the healthiest food that's delicious and incredibly easy to cook with. After all,

to stick to a smart meal plan, rule number one is not to get bored, and these balanced ingredients should keep you on your toes (promise!).

You will find something that all these healthy eating foods have in common: each is a simple ingredient, like a grain, fruit, vegetable, or dairy product. Read No pre-packaged goods insight with a laundry list of strange-sonic ingredients. You can use this as a thumb rule when shopping if the food is every day, organic, plant-based, and comes from the grocery store's periphery (i.e., where the beef, eggs, fish, and other whole foods tend to live), you're in good shape!

Now on to a list of healthy foods. Here are some extremely wholesome foods. Most are amazingly delicious.

1. Lemons

Number one is the basic but versatile lemon. As it is medicinal citrus, it goes far beyond anything you might imagine as far as a superfood. One lemon has about 100 percent of your recommended daily vitamin C intake. The fruit is anti-inflammatory and protects the organ from the body's harmful toxins. In addition, it has citrus flavonoids that can inhibit cancer cell growth.

Each morning, if you drink a glass of warm lemon water, you set up your body for a balanced digestive system and strengthen your immune system. It also serves as a purifier for blood. Calcium, potassium, pectin food, and other nutrients are positively full to the brim. In fact, one glass of juice has under 25 calories.

2. Broccoli

Broccoli, the beautiful green plant, is one of the healthiest foods in the world.

Numerous studies have been conducted about the effect of broccoli on the body,

all with positive results. Consuming reasonable amounts of broccoli will reduce cholesterol. It could also help in reducing inflammation and reactions to allergies. Broccoli is beneficial to the health of the bone and heart and helps to alkalize the body.

Quest for more? It also has a lot of kaempferol, isothiocyanates, omega-3 fatty acids. Since broccoli contains glucoraphanin and indole-3-carbinols, it may help to prevent some cancers in the body from growing. Let's eat lots more broccoli.

3. Salmon

Salmon is well known as a wholesome fish. Because of its high omega-3 benefits, it is one of the go-to fish for your inflammatory illness. It does more than assist with inflammatory disease, however. You get so much more in a piece of salmon caught young, wild.

It also contains selenium, calcium, iodine, and potassium, high on the scale of vitamin B12, D, B3, and B6. It is, therefore, perfect for bones and joints, but also for the symptoms of the brain and neurology. Cardiovascular health, improved eyesight, and smoother skin are more health benefits when you eat salmon.

4. Spinach

Spinach is more common in the average American diet these days than it was 40 years ago; that's a very good thing. It is one of the most healthy and nutritious foods you can possibly eat. Spinach has low fat and low cholesterol content. It also has a high protein and fiber content, zinc and iron, niacin, calcium, iron, magnesium, copper potassium, manganese, and vitamin-fortified. Plus, hi flavonoids!

The leafy green is filled with good things for the stomach, brain, cardiovascular, and blood pressure systems.

Oh, it's very flexible! Do some testing, and you will see that in a number of hot and cold dishes, spinach works. Popeye wasn't wrong here; it will actually help you grow big and strong.

5. Beans

A legume, or bean, is a member of the pea family, a vegetable grown in a crop that has edible seed or pod. The advice for a healthy body is that you eat about 3 cups of legumes a week, which is not that hard to really do.

We are made of protein, soluble as well as insoluble, so say hello to a healthy digestive system. Beans are low on the glycemic index, which maintains healthy blood sugar levels. It also has a good effect on heart health, cardiovascular system, blood pressure regulation, and nervous system functioning. Yet beware of beans; they're perfect for you, but don't overdo it. To help the seeds along, you should drink plenty of water.

6. Nuts

Nuts are ideal snacks and are tasty, versatile, and easy to eat. They're great for you, particularly unsalted, but not all nuts can give you all you need. These often have high levels of fat and calories. Such facts may, however, outweigh the good things that come from eating nuts in your diet. For starters, depending on the type of nut, you get fiber, potassium and zinc, vitamins A and E, and more.

What are the best ones to add to your eating plan for the week? Pistachios, hazelnuts, almonds, cashews, Nuts from Brazil, and walnuts. Macadamia and pecans are not suitable for your diet but are otherwise beneficial. Peanuts are detrimental to health but good for your brain. Any nuts you eat, nuts are unsalted, raw, young. Stay away from dried nuts or fried with salt or oil.

7. Avocados

Many people love healthy guacamole,

 but it's so much more than a dip that avocados can get in! We are a part of the berry family, incredibly good for you, and delicious. You are going to want to include consuming them in your eating plan immediately.

The avocados have up to 20 minerals and vitamins. We have low sugar and high fiber. Eating them will make you fill up faster and feel full. For sure, as they are high in fat and calories, but it is the healthy monounsaturated fat. Your consumption will be excellent so long as you don't gorge on them.

8. Garlic

Garlic comes from the family of onions and is used to improve flavor in most dishes. It's often used to aid food taste. Nevertheless, garlic contains a high quantity of a compound of sulfur called allicin, which is responsible for most of the health benefits of eating garlic.

When a garlic clove is crushed, sliced, or chewed, it produces allicin and gets to work. Garlic is a natural cold relief known to have. It can also reduce blood pressure, battle heart disease and Alzheimer's, and help you live longer.

9. Sweet Potatoes

You'd better eat sweet potato than eat an ordinary potato. The sweet potato glycemic index is much lower, and the nutritional profile is higher than that of a standard potato. We promote healthy skin, low levels of cholesterol, and properties of prostate health and cancer.

Sweet potatoes are the world's top crop for the consumption of vitamin A. We contain high vitamin C and B6 levels, and plenty of potassium. Gluten-free desserts are also a perfect way to replace carbs in a diet if you cut our potatoes or all the gluten.

10. Berries

Berries are beautiful, and so, so good to you. They have high levels of phytochemicals, which are nutrients that occur naturally to aid cell damage and overall health. Strawberries, raspberries, and blackberries are all bombs of great flavors to consume. Blueberries hit it out of the park as they have an exceptionally high antioxidant material.

Because of the benefits of brain health, eating berries can keep you mentally sharp and avoid mental degeneration; they can help control weight, fight diabetes, and keep your blood pressure down. We are also perfect for cardiac health.

Ten Naturally Antioxidant Foods

In order to stay healthy, the body needs free radicals as well as antioxidants. Nonetheless, you run the risk of conflict when one or the other is threatened. Antioxidants usually need to be replenished with high-quantity foods that contain them. This is because they don't waste free radicals too easily. Your antioxidants can likewise succumb to an event called oxidative damage. When you're low on this essential chemical, accelerated aging, broken-down tissue, cell damage, and harmful DNA content activation tend to cause you to ache. You must ingest foods high in antioxidants to avoid this auto-destruction.

1. Sumac Bran

The number in the brackets reflects this food's ORAC value, which has been in use in Middle Eastern culture as a salt supplement for centuries. ORAC stands for Radical Absorption Capability of Oxygen. People say antioxidant products, as they increase oxidant production; they also accumulate radicals and inhibit their output.

Sumac bran is the champion of antioxidant properties, almost invincible.

Although this grass is technically a spice, for various nutrients, you can eat its most natural form; that makes it a superfood.

2. Dark Chocolate

Studies say the average US resident eats approximately 12 pounds of chocolate each year. The global annual budget for chocolate is about $75 million somewhere. Seeing how everyone prefers "normal" chocolate, assuming people spend only about $5 million or less on dark chocolate is safe.

Researchers fail to understand why, as this superfood is both tasty and an unbelievable radical repellent. With an ORAC score of 21,000, dark chocolate has gone well with the junk food. Not only does dark chocolate, unlike regular chocolate, boost heart function, cholesterol levels, weight loss, cognitive function, and blood pressure.

3. Black Raspberries

Black raspberries in the United States are a bit difficult to get by. There's less space for this incredibly healthy fruit, with all the fruits, nuts, and vegetables that keep pouring into the stalls. Like red ones, there is a much higher percentage of antioxidant properties in black raspberries; they are more faithful to the taste.

Black framboises are filled with ellagic acid, gallic acid, and rutin. These are all essential phenolic compounds. Therefore, the reasons are quite obvious, the black raspberry is called the "king of berries." Some of the actual research shows that black raspberries can suppress numerous cancers and even reverse them.

4. Pecans

Pecans are a somewhat controversial superfood that has yet to have an impact on the health market.

Taking it into account the fact that this is the fourth most potent antioxidant superfood, it becomes absurd not to include it in a healthy meal plan.

Apart from the incredible 17,000 ORAC, pecans also have several other reasons to be a superfood. We are, for example, an abundant source of healthy unsaturated fat, which is doing wonders in lowering high cholesterol. These contain more than 19 minerals, including A, B, C, folic acid, magnesium, potassium, calcium, phosphorus, and zinc.

5. Elderberries

Elderberries are one of the oldest fruits known to mankind, with evidence dating from 10,000 BC. Recipes have first appeared in ancient Egypt like elderberries, while some scholars trace it back to Hippocrates. Due to the immense reach of its healing properties, the father of medicine has described this fruit as his "medicine chest."

Also shown in 1995 was the benign influence of the elderberry fruit, when the government enforced its use to combat the Panama flu epidemic. The only difference between then and now is that we know this amazing fruit's antioxidant value today; its healing dominance remains unchanged.

6. Wild Blueberries

Wild blueberries are native to northern regions of North America, unlike the cultivated blueberries. These can only be grown on North American soil, along with concord grapes and cranberries. Yet its nutritional value is needed all over the world. Luckily, wild blueberries are the resilient fruit that they are easy to grow and sustain.

Wild blueberries, along with 9,600 ORACs, contribute to many health improvements.

The tremendous amount of anthocyanin it contains makes it the best addition to every morning yogurt.

Wild blueberries are also completely cold-resistant, meaning they don't lose any nutritional value in the freezer.

7. Cranberries

Cranberries are best known for their antioxidant properties, as well as being body wide inflammation stoppers. Scientists also have reason to believe that cranberries prevent infection-inducing bacteria from binding themselves to urinary tract walls. This notion, along with their potent combination of different vitamins like C, E, and K, makes cranberries easily a superfood. These are also rich in dietary fiber, manganese, copper and pantothenic acid.

This fruit is incredibly low in calories-just 46 per cup full. In any diet which integrates cranberries, potassium and sodium establish an electrolyte balance. These also contain various anti-cancer properties. But the most potent phytonutrient of cranberries is quercetin, which contains very few berries in this quantity.

8. Kidney Beans

Kidney beans are the only non-sweet food to make this list, in addition to pecans. They contain high amounts of fibers, which reduces bad cholesterol significantly. The fiber-rich content often negates the increase in blood sugar levels after a meal; this notion is an extremely beneficial feature for all diabetes-induced people. What makes kidney beans special on the list is their super-high molybdenum content, a trace mineral that detoxifies sulfites.

Because sulfites are a food-preservative that is commonly found in any salad, there is almost no meal that can't compliment the kidney beans. This food was once native to Peru, but it spread rapidly throughout the rest of the world. Consequently, kidney beans are now among the cheapest superfoods on the market.

9. Prunes

Dried plums make one of the most potent laxatives of nature, owing to their high sorbitol content. It makes prunes an old traditional remedy for constipation and other digestive problems. This fruit has a high sugar content, which is very low in calories (only 30 per piece), making them a great addition to any diet.

Also present in prunes are the phytonutrients called phenols, which are present in most superfoods. That ingredient gives them a high ranking of antioxidants. The fruit also contains a high amount of soluble fibers; they are responsible for making you feel much fuller after a meal. It, in effect, avoids overheating and improves the conditions associated with weight.

10. Black Currant

Because of the myth that black currant spreads the disease that destroys pine trees, it took a long time for US farmers to know the extent of benefits this superfood provides. Luckily, the United States finally lifted the ban, and we can now fully enjoy the full potential and positivity of this delicious fruit.

Black currant is definitely an excellent source of anthocyanin's, polyphenolic compounds, gamma-linoleic acid, and vitamin C. The British seem to be particularly aware of these attributes since they have integrated this food into many nutritious meals and drinks across the UK. Black currant tartness makes it an excellent addition to any jelly, juice, or smoothie.

3.2 Herbs

Herbs are the leaf component of a plant that can be used fresh or dried in the cooking process.

Any other component of the herb,

typically dried, is called spice. These include bark (cinnamon), berries (peppercorns), seeds (cumin), roots (turmeric), flower (chamomile), buds (cloves), and a flower's stigma (saffron), for example.

Herbs are a finest way to add flavor and color to any kind of sweet or savory dish or drink without adding fat, salt, or sugar. We do appear to have their own range of health-promoting properties in addition to taste and color.

In general, fresh herbs are seasoned delicately, so in the last few minutes, if you add them to your cooking, do so. Degustation of your dish as you walk along will help you tell whether you added enough. If insufficient herbs are used, then the flavor of the dish will make little difference, but if too many herbs are used, their flavor will overshadow other ingredients.

Health benefits of herbs

Herbal consumption can help prevent and control heart disease, cancer, and diabetes. It can also help to reduce blood clots and provide anti-inflammatory properties as well as anti-tumor. Work is still ongoing, but studies have shown that:

• Garlic, linseed, fenugreek, and lemongrass can help to reduce cholesterol levels.

• Garlic is good for those with moderately high blood pressure.

• Fenugreek can help control the activity of blood sugar and insulin (as can linseed, flaxseed, and cinnamon).

• Garlic, onions, chives, leeks, mint, basil, oregano, sage, and many other herbs can aid in cancer protection.

• Herbs are rich in antioxidants, particularly cloves, cinnamon, sage, oregano, and thyme, helping to reduce lipoproteins in low density (' bad' cholesterol).

Fresh herbs often have higher levels of antioxidants compared to processed or dried herbs, but if you use herbs to leverage their health-promoting qualities first and foremost, try to add your fresh herbs at the end of the cooking or to preserve them.

10 Herbs and Spices with the most Health Benefits

People worldwide have learned about the healing power of herbs and spices for decades. Here's the science behind why they're so amazing for you, and advice on how to get their fill. A cinnamon sprinkle on your morning coffee. A sprinkle of basil, finely sliced over pasta. You know how just about any meal will wake up herbs and spices. But they can do a lot to keep you safe too. Here are some of our favorite herbs ' health benefits and spices-plus tasty ways of using them. Many herbs can cause side effects in large doses or interfere with medications. Using caution and tell your doctor what herbal supplements you are taking.

Historically the use of herbs and spices has been incredibly important. Some, well before culinary use, were praised for their medicinal properties. Modern science has now shown that there are indeed significant health benefits for many of them. Here are 10 of the healthiest herbs and spices in the world that are backed by studies.

1. Cinnamon has a Powerful Anti-Diabetic Effect

Cinnamon is one of the popular spices found in recipes and baked goods of all kinds. This contains a compound called cinnamaldehyde, which accounts for the medicinal properties of cinnamon. Cinnamon has strong antioxidant activity, helps fight inflammation, and has been shown to decrease blood cholesterol and triglycerides. But the effect of cinnamon on blood sugar levels is where it really shines.

Cinnamon can reduce blood sugar by several mechanisms,

including by slowing down carbohydrate breakdown in the digestive tract and improving insulin sensitivity.

Research has shown that cinnamon in diabetic patients, which is a significant amount, can reduce fasting blood sugars by 10-29 percent. Usually, the effective dose is 0.5-2 teaspoons of cinnamon a day, or 1-6 grams. Cinnamon has many health benefits and is particularly effective in minimizing blood-sugar levels.

2. Sage Can Improve Brain Function

Sage drives its name from the Latin word Salvere, meaning "to save." During the Middle Ages, she had a strong reputation for her healing properties and was even used to help prevent the plague. Current research suggests that sage can enhance brain function and memory, particularly in people with Alzheimer's disease. A decrease in the amount of acetylcholine, a chemical messenger in the brain, causes Alzheimer's disease. Sage hinders acetylcholine degradation.

A 4-month study of 42 people with mild to moderate Alzheimer's disease showed that sage extract produces significant improvements in brain function. Other studies also showed that sage could enhance memory function in healthy people, young and old alike. There is a promising evidence that sage extract can improve the function of brain and memory, especially in people with disease like Alzheimer's.

3. Peppermint Relieves IBS Pain

Peppermint holds a very long history of use in Folk and Aromatherapy medicine. As with many herbs, it is the oily component which contains the agents responsible for the effects on the health. Several studies have shown that peppermint oil in irritable bowel syndrome, or IBS, can improve pain management. It seems to work by calming the colon's smooth muscles, which relieves the pain experienced during bowel movements. It also helps in the reduction of abdominal bloating, a common digestive symptom.

There are also studies that show peppermint can help fight

nausea in aromatherapy. Peppermint aromatherapy caused significant reductions in nausea in a study of over 1,100 women in labor. Nausea following surgery and C-section births have also been shown to decrease. The natural peppermint oil provides pain relief for those with IBS. When used in aromatherapy, it also has potent anti-nausea effects.

4. Turmeric Contains a Substance with Powerful Anti-Inflammatory Effects

Turmeric is the spice that gives its yellow color to the curry. It contains several medicinally characterized compounds, the most important of which is curcumin. Curcumin is a remarkably powerful antioxidant that helps to combat oxidative damage and boosts the body's own antioxidant enzymes. This is important because it is believed that oxidative damage is one of the key mechanisms behind aging and many diseases. Curcumin is also highly anti-inflammatory, to the extent that it matches the effectiveness of certain anti-inflammatory drugs. Given that long-term, low-level inflammation plays a vital role in almost any chronic Western illness, and it is not shocking to see that curcumin is associated with a range of benefits to health.

Studies suggest it can enhance brain function, fight Alzheimer's, reduce the risk of heart disease and cancer, and relieve arthritis, to name but a few. Here's a post about turmeric/curcumin's many amazing health benefits. Research has shown that curcumin, the active ingredient in turmeric spice, has significant benefits for many health aspects.

5. Holy Basil Helps Fight Infections and raise Immunity

The holy basil is considered a sacred herb in India, not to be confused with standard basil or Thai basil. Studies show that holy basil can prevent a number of bacteria, yeasts, and molds from growing in. One small study also found that by growing certain immune cells in the blood, it can improve immune system function.

Holy basil is also associated with reduced levels of blood sugar before and after meals, as well as with the treatment of depression related to anxiety. Such studies were fairly small, however, and more research is needed before any recommendations can be made. Holy basil tends to boost the immune function and to suppress bacteria, yeasts, and mold growth.

6. Cayenne Pepper have Anti-Cancer Properties

Cayenne pepper is a kind of chili pepper that is used for making spicy dishes. Capsaicin is the active ingredient in it, which has been shown in many studies to suppress appetite and improve fat burning. For this reason, in many commercial weight-loss drugs, it is a common ingredient. One of the studies found that adding 1 gram of red pepper to meals reduced appetite and increased the burning of fat in people who did not consume peppers regularly. There was absolutely no effect in people who were accustomed to eating spicy food, however, indicating that a tolerance to the effects could build up.

Several animal studies have found capsaicin to fight other forms of cancer, including cancer of the lungs, liver, and prostate. Of course, these anticancer effects that have been observed are far from being confirmed in humans, so take all of this with a big salt. Cayenne pepper is very rich in capsaicin, a substance that reduces appetite and boosts fat burning. It also showed potential for anticancer generally in animal based studies.

7. Ginger has Anti-Inflammatory Properties

In several forms of alternative medicine, ginger is a popular spice. Research has repeatedly shown that nausea can be successfully treated with 1 gram or more of ginger. This includes nausea from morning sickness, chemotherapy, and sea disease.

Ginger also seems to have strong anti-inflammatory properties and can help manage pain. One research in subjects at risk for colon cancer showed that markers for colon inflammation decreased by 2 grams of ginger extract per day in the same way as aspirin. Other research found that those with osteoarthritis reported a combination of ginger, cinnamon, mastic, and sesame oil reduced pain and stiffness. It has had a comparable effect to aspirin or ibuprofen therapy. For many forms of nausea, 1 gram of ginger seems to be an effective treatment. It is anti-inflammatory as well and can help reduce pain.

8. Fenugreek Improves Blood Sugar Control

Fenugreek was commonly used in Ayurveda, especially for libido and masculinity enhancement. While its effects are inconclusive on testosterone levels, fenugreek does appear to have beneficial effects on blood sugar. It contains the 4-hydroxy isoleucine plant protein, which can improve the hormone insulin function. Several human studies have shown that, especially in diabetics, at least 1 gram of fenugreek extract per day can lower blood sugar levels. It has been shown that fenugreek enhances insulin regulation, leading to significant amount of reductions in blood-sugar proportions.

9. Rosemary Can Help Prevent Allergies

Rosemary's active ingredient is called rosmarinic acid. This substance has been shown to alleviate allergic reactions and nasal congestion. In a 29-person test, rosmarinic acid doses of both 50 and 200 mg were shown to relieve allergy symptoms. The number of immune cells also decreased in nasal mucus, with reduced congestion. Rosmarinic acid has anti-inflammatory effects that seem to suppress symptoms of allergy and help reduce the nasal congestions.

10. Garlic Improve Heart Health

The primary use of garlic over the course of ancient history was for its medicinal properties. We very well know that most of these health effects derive from a compound called allicin, which is also responsible for the distinct scent of garlic. Garlic intake, like a common cold, is well known for reducing sickness. If you get cold sometimes, then adding more garlic to your diet might be incredibly helpful.

Evidence for beneficial effects on heart health is also convincing. Ail supplementation tends to reduce total and/or LDL cholesterol by about 10-15 percent for those with high cholesterol. Human studies have also found garlic intake in people with high blood pressure to cause significant decreases in blood pressure. For one study, it was just as effective as a medication that reduces the blood pressure.

3.3 Strategizing your diet plan

While switching to a healthy diet doesn't have to be a decision about everything or nothing. You just don't have to be perfect, you don't have to remove things that you love absolutely, and you don't have to adjust everything at once — which usually leads to cheating or giving up on your new eating plan.

It would be a better approach to make a few minor changes at a time. Maintaining modest goals will help you achieve more in the long run without feeling deprived or stressed by a big diet overhaul. Think of preparing a healthy diet as a set of small, manageable steps— like adding salad once a day to your diet. When your minor changes become routine, you can keep adding healthier choices.

Setting yourself up for success

Try to keep things easy to set yourself up for success. No need to stress consuming a healthier diet.

For example, rather than being overly concerned with counting calories, think about your diet as in terms of color, variety, and freshness on the whole. Carefully focus on avoiding all types of packaged and processed foods and, where possible, opting for more fresh ingredients.

Prepare more of your meals yourself. Try cooking more meals at home will help you take over what you eat and better monitor exactly what's going on in your diet. You'll eat fewer calories and avoid chemical additives, added sugar, and unhealthy fats from packaged and take-out foods that can make you feel tired, bloated, and irritable, exacerbating symptoms of depression, stress, and anxiety.

Implement the changes right. It is important to replace these with healthy alternatives when cutting back on unhealthy foods in your diet. Replacing unhealthy trans fats with healthy fats (such as grilled chicken converting to grilled salmon) would make a positive health difference. However, switching animal fats to refined carbohydrates (such as switching a donut's breakfast bacon) won't reduce your risk of heart disease or improve your mood.

Write the protocol. It is extremely important or simply take it as mendatory for you to be aware of what is in your food as suppliers frequently conceal large amounts of sugar or unhealthy fats in packaged foods, including foods that claim to be safe.

Take a look at how you feel after eating. That will help to promote new healthy habits and tastes. The healthier a meal you eat, the better after a meal you will feel. The more you eat junk food, the more likely you will feel uncomfortable, nauseous, or drained of energy.

Soak up plenty of water. Water helps flush out waste products and toxins systems, yet many of us go through dehydrated life — causing fatigue, low energy, and headaches. It is normal to confuse hunger thirst, and staying well hydrated will also help you make healthier choices about food.

Moderation: important to any healthy diet

What exactly is moderation? Essentially it only means eating as much food as the body needs. At the end of a meal, you should feel satisfied but not stuffed. Moderation means fewer for many of us than we do now. But it does not mean that the foods you love are eliminated. For example, eating bacon once a week might be considered moderate if you follow it with a balanced lunch and dinner, but not if you would follow it with a box of sweets like donuts or a pepperoni pizza.

Try not to think of certain types of foods as totally "off-limits." It's normal to want those foods more when you ban those foods, and then feel like a failure when you cede to the temptations. Simply start by reducing portion sizes of unhealthy foods, rather than consuming them as often as possible. As you reduce to your intake of unhealthy foods, you might feel less anxious about them or think of them as indulgences only occasionally.

Speak of portions smaller. Serving sizes have recently ballooned. Choose a fine starter instead of an entrée while eating out, share a meal with a friend, and don't order something supersized. Visual hints can help with portion sizes at home. Your beef, fish, or chicken serving should be the size of a card deck, with half a cup of mashed potato, rice, or pasta about the size of a typical light bulb. You can probably trick your brain into thinking it's a bigger portion by serving your meals on smaller plates or in bowls. If you are not happy at the end of a meal, add more leafy greens or add fruit to the meal.

Grab your time. It is important to slow down and think about food as nourishment rather than just gulping in between meetings or on the way to picking up the children. It actually takes your brain a couple of minutes to convince your body it's had enough food, so eat slowly and stop eating until you feel full.

Eat whenever possible, with others. Eating alone, especially in front of a TV or a computer, often leads to a carefree overeating.

Limit homemade snack foods. Pay attention to the foods you have at hand. Eating in moderation is more difficult if you have ready-made unhealthy snacks and treatments. Alternatively, surround yourself with healthy choices and go out and get it then when you're able to reward yourself with a special treat.

Checks mental feeding. We're not always feeding purely to relieve hunger. Most of us also turn to food for stress relief or to cope with unpleasant emotions like sadness, loneliness, or boredom.

But you can regain control over the food you eat and your feelings by finding healthy ways to manage stress and emotions.

It is not just what you are consuming, but when you are fed. Eat breakfast all day, and eat smaller meals. A healthy breakfast will improve your metabolism, and eating small, healthy meals can keep your energy going all day. Avoid eating late into the evening. Try eating dinner earlier.

With Attention, add more fruit and vegetables to your routine

Fruits and vegetables are healthy, as they are low in calories and rich in nutrients, meaning they're filled with vitamins, minerals, antioxidants, and fiber.

Focus on eating at least five portions of fruit and vegetables on the recommended daily amount, and it will obviously fill you up and help you cut back on unhealthy foods. For example, a serving is half a cup of raw fruit or veg, or a little apple or banana. Many of us need to double the amount that we eat right now.

Raising your consumption:

• Add antioxidant-rich berries to your daily cereal breakfast

• Eat a medley of sweet fruit — oranges, mangos, pineapples, grapes — for dessert

• Replace your regular rice or pasta side dish for a vibrant salad

• Instead of eating processed snack foods, snacks on vegetables such as broccoli, snow peas or cherry tomatoes along with a spicy hummus dip or peanut butter.

How to make vegetables tasty?

Although plain salads and steamed veggies can easily become bland, your vegetable dishes have plenty of ways to add flavor.

Add some color. Not only do lighter, darker colored vegetables contain higher vitamin, mineral, and antioxidant concentrations, but they can also change the taste and make meals more visually appealing. Using fresh or sunny tomatoes, glazed carrots or beets, roasted red chopsticks, yellow squash, or soft, colorful peppers to add color.

Live greens of salads. Branch out lettuce beyond. Kale, arugula, spinach, mustard greens, broccoli, and nutrient-packed Chinese cabbage try chopping with olive oil, adding a spicy dressing, or sprinkling with slices of almond, chickpeas, a little bacon, parmesan or goat cheese to add flavor to your salad greens.

Has your sweet tooth fulfilled? Sweet vegetables, of course—such as carrots, beets, sweet potatoes, yams, onions, bell peppers, and squash add sweetness to your meals and reduce your cravings for added sugar. For a satisfying sweet kick, add them to soups, stews, or pasta sauces.

Cook in new ways green beans, broccoli, sprouts from Brussels, and asparagus. Avoid grilling, roasting, or frying them with chili flakes, onions, shallots, mushrooms, or onion rather than boiling or steaming these balanced sides. Until serving, marinate in tangy lemon or lime.

Plan quick and easy meals ahead

Eating healthy begins with great planning. If you have a well-stocked kitchen, quick and easy recipes, and plenty of healthy snacks, you'll have won half the healthy diet battle.

1. Design your meals by the sevens or even the thirties

This is arguably one of the best ways to have a healthy diet is to prepare and eat your own food regularly. Choose some healthy recipes you and your family like and build a meal plan around them. If you have three or four meals scheduled per week and eat the rest of the nights, you'll be farther ahead than eating out or having frozen dinners most nights.

2. Shop the perimeter of the grocery store

Healthy eating products are generally found around the outer edges of most grocery stores, while the middle aisles are lined with refined and packed foods that are not good for you. Go and shop the perimeter of the store for most of your food (fresh fruit and vegetables, fish and poultry, whole-grain breads and dairy products), add a few items from the freezer section (frozen fruits and vegetables), and visit the aisles for spices, oils, and whole grains (such as rolled oats, brown rice, whole-wheat pasta).

3. Cook when you can

Try to cook one or both weekend or weekend nights and add extra to freeze or set aside for a different night. Cooking ahead saves time and money, and it's gratifying to know you've got a home-cooked meal waiting for you to eat.

Stand up and challenge yourself to come up with two or three recipes that you can put together without going to the store — using stuff in your cupboard, freezer, and spice rack. A delicious, whole grain pasta dinner with a fast tomato sauce or a quick and easy black bean quesadilla on a whole wheat flour tortilla (among countless other recipes) might serve as your go-to meal when you're too busy for shopping or cooking.

Diet Plans

It is not difficult to plan a daily diet as long as each meal and snack has some protein, fiber, complex carbohydrates, and some fat. Here's what every meal you need to say.

Eating breakfast lets, you get plenty of energy to start your day. Don't ruin your breakfast with foods high in fat and high in calories. For your breakfast, choose some protein and fiber, and it's a good time to eat some fresh fruit.

Completely optional mid-morning snack. Whether you eat a bigger breakfast, you may not feel hungry until midday. Nonetheless, whether you feel a bit hungry and lunch is still two or three hours away, a small snack in the middle of the morning will tide you over without adding many calories.

Lunch is often something you eat at work or at school, so it's a perfect time to pack a sandwich or leftovers you can heat up. Or choose a balanced, clear soup and fresh veggie salad if you buy your lunch.

Also, an optional a mid-afternoon snack. Keep it low in calories and consume enough to hold you from getting too hungry, because dinner is only a few hours away.

Dinner is a time when over-eating is easy, particularly if you haven't eaten much during the day, so watch your serving sizes. Cut your plate into four quarters mentally. One-fourth is for your meat or protein source, one-fourth is for a starch and the last two-fourths are for fresh and colorful vegetables or green salad.

A lightweight, carbohydrate-rich evening snack may help you sleep, but avoid hard, greasy foods or high-sugar foods.

5 Diets That Are Supported by Science

While many diets can work for you, the key is to find one that you like and be able to stick to long-term. Here are five healthy diets that have been scientifically proven successful.

1. Low-carb, whole-food diet

The low-carb, whole-food diet is perfect for people who need to lose weight, improve their wellbeing, and raising their disease risk. It is versatile, allowing you to fine-tune your carb intake according to your goals. This diet is high in vegetables, meat, fish, eggs, berries, nuts, and fats but low in starch, sugars, and processed foods.

2. Mediterranean diet

The Mediterranean diet has been thoroughly studied and is an outstanding diet. It's especially effective for preventing heart disease. This highlights foods that were widely eaten around the Mediterranean world during the 20th and earlier centuries. It contains plenty of vegetables, fruits, fish, poultry, whole grains, legumes, dairy products, and olive oil extra virgin.

3. Paleo diet

The paleo diet is a very common diet that is effective for weight loss and enhancement of the general health.

At the moment, it is the most common diet in the world. It focuses on unprocessed foods, which are thought to imitate those available to some of the Paleolithic ancestors of humanity.

4. Vegan diet

In the past decade, the vegan diet has become more and more popular. It is associated with a number of health benefits, including weight loss, heart health enhancement, and better control of blood sugar. The diet is based on plant foods solely and excludes all animal products.

5. Gluten-free diet

The gluten-free diet is important for people who have a gluten allergy, a protein found in wheat, rye, and barley. You will concentrate on whole foods that are naturally gluten-free for optimum health. Gluten-free junk food also contains junk food.

The bottom line is this

So many diets exist that simply finding a single one to try can feel overwhelming. It is extremely important for you to note, however, that certain eating habits have more scientific support than others. Whether you want to lose weight or actually improve your overall health, try to find diets that are research-supported.

3.4 Major benefits

A well-balanced diet offers all the energy you need to keep active throughout the day, plus the nutrients you need to develop and repair, helping you stay active and healthy, and help prevent diet-related diseases, like some cancers. Maintaining active and eating a healthy, balanced diet can also help you stay healthy.

20 Benefits of healthy eating

Most people perceive healthy diets as boring, and they don't want to change their eating habits until they have a health problem or become overweight.

Whatever the current diet view may be, the following 20 healthy eating advantages are sufficiently inspiring to begin paying more attention to what to eat.

1. Improved Mood and Mental Health

Perhaps this one is the most satisfying. We just want to feel good, after all. A proper nutrient-rich diet, particularly B vitamins, antioxidants, and healthy fats, will nurture your brain and balance the mood-regulating neurotransmitters. Some probiotic strains might even help with mild depression, anxiety, and other mental disorders.

2. Increased Energy Levels

Feeling fatigued after each meal? Refined sugar, processed meat, and fast food should be blamed for this. Processed sugar will give you a quick rush of energy, but it will actually make your exhaustion worse over the long term. Whole fruits, seeds, and nuts naturally raise your stamina and hold you up all day long.

3. Reduced Stress

Psychological and environmental factors play an essential role in managing stress, but a healthy diet can also calm you down. It keeps the levels of cortisol (the stress hormone) under control and avoids vast swings in blood sugar, which may cause stress. One of the easiest ways to relax is to drink a warm cup of herbal tea. Some healthy foods such as bananas, pistachios, and avocado can also aid.

4. Weight Control

The Obesity rates in developed, and developing countries are skyrocketing

; a sedentary lifestyle and overconsumption of junk food are the two major causes. A healthy diet will most certainly keep your weight under control and will make you fit, beautiful and confident. Of course, you should try to stay healthy and do more to achieve optimum results.

5. Better Sleep

Do not consider eating right in front of your bed. Simply give your belly a few hours of rest before you sleep, and hold warm for your dinners. New salads will provide you with plenty of nutrients without overloading; good sources of magnesium such as spinach, nuts, and seeds are especially welcome.

6. Optimal Hydration

The best and easy way to stay hydrated is to drink more water. Who'd have guessed?? Apart from kidding, a healthy diet also leads to maximum hydration, which is crucial to everything! A diet rich in fresh fruit and veggies provides plenty of oxygen.

Limiting sugar and salt intake is essential because they can' bury' water and dry you out. The water that you drink matters, too. Bottled water is fantastic, and tap water is just as good as having a good source. If not, then investment in a water filtration system may be worthwhile.

7. Cleaner Skin

"Beauty comes from within" is true also for your skin. Proper hydration and a balanced diet will ensure your looks are kept smooth and rejuvenated. Good sources of Omega-3 such as flaxseed, walnuts, and fatty fish deserve special consideration.

8. Staying Active and Fit

Healthy eating helps you keep your weight optimal, and keeps you energized. Then you move naturally towards an active lifestyle and enjoy staying fit. This is a vicious cycle.

9. Prevent Diseases

Now one thing is for sure, after decades of detailed research: food and lifestyle patterns play a central role in disease prevention. A healthy diet will reduce the risk of illness and pain, from cancer and heart disease to skin ulcers and headaches (and everything else in between). As this saying goes, "a healthy person has a thousand wishes, and only one for a sick person" A 10-minute headache is all it takes to remember how important good health is. Do your utmost to preserve it.

10. Cure Diseases

"Let food be your medicine, and let medicine be your food."-Hippocrates This one is now a bit controversial. While western allopathic medicine still holds chemical drugs as their' holy grail' of healing, functional medicine is practiced by a growing number of health experts.

Instead of coping with symptoms, the particular holistic approach addresses the root cause of diseases. Naturally, nutrition plays a central role in this approach and builds the foundations for every healing process.

11. Live Longer

I like to focus on quality over quantity, but if you extend your lifespan, you've been covered again by a healthy diet. This one is closely related to the two previous advantages. Most of the deaths are caused by heart disease, cancer, and diabetes, especially in the US and European countries.

Given that healthy eating can help prevent these diseases, and even cure them, the effect on longevity becomes apparent. Studies have shown that specific diets, such as DASH and Mediterranean, are essential to survival.

12. Age Better

Healthy eating and daily exercise benefits= fresh skin + health

+ avoidance of illness + longevity + clarity of mind= an alchemical recipe for healthy aging. And who wouldn't want to survive the ravages of time?

Invest in a healthy diet and lifestyle before investing money on expensive anti-aging products and treatments. Moderate limits on calories can also extend the lifespan and even reverse aging.

13. Increase Your Productivity and Attention

Do your dietary choices affect the performance of your work/school? There is a strong connection between nutrition and productivity, a poor diet with lots of sugar and processed junk food will result in:

• Tiredness and irritability

• Reduced energy levels

• Increased stress levels

• Poor mental concentration

Healthy eating will help you to conquer this state of affairs and keep your performance sound. Nutrients that can increase your productivity include:

• Folate (leafy greens, whole grains, and beans)

• Omega-3 fatty acids (fatty fish, flaxseeds, walnuts, hemp seeds)

• Antioxidants (beers and citrus fruits, greens and nuts)

14. Optimal Growth and Development of Teenagers

The nutritional benefits already listed are even more important for a developing body and mind. You are still physically developing as a teenager and need all of the essential nutrients to build a strong, healthy body.

Sadly, for healthy eating, teens do not always pay much attention.

Think twice, and good dietary habits will help improve your looks, confidence, attitude, and grades, thanks to all of the benefits mentioned. Developing healthy eating habits can support you throughout your life, and help you enjoy more positive experiences in your life. Can you give veggies a try?

15. Eat More and Enjoy Food

No, you don't need to weigh every single bite. Once you know the basic rules and start eating real nutrient-dense food, you won't get any benefit from a few more servings. You shouldn't be afraid of binge eating on a healthy diet, and it's usually associated with unhealthy junk food and bad dieting habits.

Did you ever see someone gorge on apples? Sure, healthy food will taste great, and you'll still love to eat. It's something you get used to and appreciate more with the passing of time. Pick dark chocolate, nut butter, or a homemade ice cream and learn how to make delicious full-food meals.

16. Save Money

Wait, don't all argue that healthy food costs a lot more? This depends on what you mean by, and what you equate with,' healthy diet.' When you cook your own meals, and don't overdo exotic ingredients, on a budget you can eat healthy. It can cost you even less than surviving on pizzas, hamburgers, French fries and snacks that are purchased from the supermarket. Another perfect way to save money and change your diet is by cutting meat.

A diet based on plants provides many healthy eating advantages, and the basic ingredients are generally cheaper than meat. When you incorporate long-term savings from disease prevention and increased productivity of work, a healthy diet can save you a lot of money.

17. Inspire others

Any change in your attitudes and habits, whether positive or negative, is affecting people around you.

 Instead of letting others ' bad dietary choices influence your diet and health, make a positive change and encourage them to keep up. You don't have to preach healthy eating and accuse those who don't care about it, which just irritates everyone.

Your actions will, of course, move people who care about you and admire you. Once you start preparing healthy meals, invite and encourage your friends to try some of the recipes.

18. Raise Healthier and Smarter Kids

If you start eating right, you'll feed your children well and encourage them to follow the same habits as they grow up. In every stage of child development, proper nutrition is important starting from a mother's diet during pregnancy. Food acts as knowledge, and influences our DNA, according to the latest studies. Your dietary choices influence your genes directly and shape your offspring's health.

19. Save the Environment

What if I told you how much food you buy and eat would decide the entire planet's future? Factory farming is one of the most important causes of:

• Air, water, and land contamination

• Water shortages

• Deforestation

• Biodiversity loss

In other words, it destroys our climate. In making smart dietary choices that ultimately protect your health and our world, you will help to end that. Cut back on animal products and pick organic alternatives from sustainable local farms focused on pasture. Even if you buy packaged foods or snacks, you lead to plastic pollution, one of the greatest environmental problems we face.

20. Positive Social and Ethical Impact

Whatever our dietary choices, we're all spending a lot of our money on food. Have you ever considered the social and ethical implications of that money? Each buck you invest causes a supply and demand chain reaction.

Many farms treat both livestock and farm workers appallingly. Farm workers often suffer pesticide poisoning in conventional agriculture. The giant food companies also demand hard labor for a lower than average wage. On the other hand, local organic farms tend to pay more attention to farmworkers, animal welfare, and the environment.

You're expecting different actions and behaviors when buying products from various sources. Money is a double edge sword; make sure that you use it correctly. Do not think of a healthy diet as something bland, which is intended for people with health and weight problems. Every single aspect of your life will profit and bring many positive changes. The list merely highlights the most obvious and significant advantages, although I have probably left out many more that are worth mentioning.

Hopefully, this will inspire you to change your health and take a closer look at what you eat.

Chapter 4: Stress Management is the key

Stress management plays a vital role with regard to health in our lives. One who is able to cope with stress will easily boost health. In this chapter, the riddle of handling stress can be opened and addressed through exploration, awareness and solution to conquer stress and start living a healthy life.

In our lives, we all experience stress. Because the vast majority of health issues are triggered or affected by stress, recognizing how stress affects your body and practicing successful stress management strategies is important to make stress work for you rather than against you.

What Is Stress?

Stress is the reaction of your body to your life changes. Since life involves constant change (from moving places from home to work every morning to adjusting to big changes in life such as a loved one's marriage, divorce, or death), there is no escaping stress. This is why the goal should not be to remove all stress but to eliminate unnecessary stress and handle the rest effectively. Some people experience some common causes of stress, but each person is different.

Always know a good laugh has a way to lighten your burdens? Perhaps you've encountered one such situation. Your day feels totally stressful and overwhelming, but then you're coaching yourself to step away from the frenzy, collect your thoughts, list what's going on–prioritizing

 what's important. Has your list ever helped you find that your day might be more and easily manageable compared to it seemed? Or just maybe you usually go walking with a friend before beginning your day at work.

This week seems too crazy and exhausting to fit into such "frivolities," so you decide you're going to go ahead and walk instead of missing it. You also find that it was beneficial for you mentally, socially, and emotionally, and you actually feel more able to attack the task list when you sit down for the workday.

Learn to stress-pump the brakes. Laughter, physical activity and organizing of your thinking can be powerful methods of stress management. But something as simple as a brief break can be successful, too. Dr. Robert Sapolsky, Stanford stress specialist and professor of neurology, says we all need to devote ourselves to daily stress management and learn how to "pump the brakes" on stress without pushing it onto others. Let's think about why and how.

What is the objective of the stress? Emotions are signals which help us to recognize issues. Stress hormones help us fight or flee when at risk. But the stress response of our body can become a concern if it continuously suggests danger over problems that aren't actually a threat or if it develops to the point of overwhelming our health, well-being or clear thinking.

How to practice handling stress? Your mind deserves better than thinking about being weighed down with the never-ending work! Some stress can be helpful and can actually solve problems, but much of our stress is needless and even harmful. It is clear that stressed brains do not function in the same manner as unstressed brains.

How do we exactly learn to manage our stress?

Step 1: Awareness! Learn about your Low Zone.

Stress has a tendency to become chronic when daily life's stresses weigh down on us.

Or maybe in your life,

you've become accustomed to stress and allow anything that

 is actually the most stressful topic to decide what you're going to do every day. Everyone in their lives wants fun, efficiency and innovation and chronic stress robs us of these.

Look at this continuum: I'm interested in living, creatively, and cheerfully. I'm comfortable and this is how I expect to stay. I can deal with tension and think about the constructive answers to my problems. I am somewhat irritable, nervous, or depressed and I feel stressed. My problems are seemingly insoluble. I get annoyed or disturbed by many things. Help! Help! I'm going to lose them! I've had chart-topping negative feelings.

How are you now putting yourself? How do you know when the moderate point is passed? Identify for yourself the small changes in your mood that you can feel when you step up the continuum. This may take a few days to look at yourself, but if you're like most people (and you're likely to be good!), the stress level will rise in a predictable pattern. When you take time to learn your emotional signs, you can learn how to control your stress, so you can spend more time in the "weak zone."

But you have no idea how hard my life is! Clearly, some people have more stressful experiences than others, and unless they learn to manage stress and improve their quality of life, those people will probably pay a toll for it. For example, the burden of becoming a caregiver also results in emotional health problems and health difficulties. If you are a caregiver, it is particularly important that you develop stress management skills so that you can remain in the "low zone," find ways to enjoy your life and have moments of happiness and joy in your care.

Step 2: Try to Live in the Low Zone.

Once you have passed the mid-zone mark into the high-stress

zone, it is time to take a moment of stress management.

 Perhaps that means you're calling a friend, taking a short five-minute outdoor stroll, knowing what you can and can't change or having a funny book on hand that you can read whenever you need a laugh. And whatever works best for you, take the time to get your stress level back closer to the "weak zone." Remember what happens when you take these breaks with your body and mind.

There are certain benefits to living in the low-zone. The benefits of living in a low zone are plentiful! You will feel more innovative, happy and capable of experiencing tiny moments of happiness. You always reserve your "high-zone stress responses" for occasions when it is more fitting to do so. If life and death are not on the table, we don't need intense chart-topping responses. Let's learn to enjoy life's blessings and put away the pressures whenever we can.

Stress basics

Stress reflects a natural psychological and physical reaction to life's demands. A small amount of stress can be beneficial and can inspire you to do well. Yet several obstacles a day can drive you beyond your ability to cope, such as sitting in traffic, meeting deadlines and paying bills.

For your defense, your brain comes with a hard-wired alarm system. Whenever your brain perceives a possible threat, your body is signaled to release a burst of hormones that will increase your heart rate and increase your blood pressure. This "fight-or-flight" response will fuel you to tackle the danger.

Once the threat is gone, the body will return to a normal, healthy condition. Unfortunately, modern life's nonstop complications mean some people's alarm systems rarely shut down.

Stress management lets you reset your alarm system with a range of tools. It can help you to adapt to your mind and body

 (resilience). Your body could always be on high alert, without it. Chronic stress can lead to severe health problems over time.

Before stress affects your health, relationships or quality of life, don't wait. Today, start practicing stress management strategies.

Stress relief

Modern life's pace and challenges make stress management necessary for all.

Next, identify the causes in order to monitor your tension. Which makes you feel frustrated, stressed, nervous, and irritable? Do you often experience headaches or an upset stomach that has no medical cause?

Some stressors are easy to identify, such as job pressures, relationship problems or financial concerns. Yet daily hassles and requests, such as long-term waiting or a late meeting, often add to your stress level.

Even events that are inherently good, such as getting married or buying a house, can be stressful. Any life-change can cause stress.

Once you've defined the stress factors, find methods to fix them. A good starting point is to recognize what you can monitor. For example, if stress dont let you sleep, the remedy can be as simple as removing your bedroom's TV and computer and letting your mind wind down before bedtime.

Some occasions, such as when stress is centered on high work demands or a loved one's illness, maybe you can only change your reaction.

Don't feel like you've got to work this out yourself. Whether you need anyone to listen to you, help with child care or a ride to work while your car is in the shop, seek help and support from family and friends.

Many people benefit from deep breathing practices, tai chi,

yoga, meditation, or being in nature. Set time aside for yourself. Get a massage, soak up in a bubble bath, dance, listen to music, watch a movie... something you can relax.

Keeping a healthy lifestyle helps you manage stress. Eat a healthy diet, do regular exercise and get enough sleep. Make a conscious effort to spend less time in front of a screen — TV, laptop, computer, and telephone — and relax more.

Stress will not go away from your life. And it has to be constant stress reduction. But you can combat some of the negative effects of stress and improve your ability to cope with difficulties by paying attention to what triggers the stress and practicing ways of relaxing.

Why is it so important to manage stress?

If you are living with high stress levels, you're putting your whole well-being at risk. Stress causes damage to your emotional balance, as well as to your physical health. This narrows your ability to think clearly, work well and enjoy life. It might sound like you can't do anything about tension. The bills won't stop coming, there will never be more hours in the day and there will always be demanding responsibilities for your work and family. You have much more power, however, than you might think.

Good stress management helps you split your life's hold tension, so you can be happier, safer, and more efficient. The ultimate goal is a healthy life, with time for work, relationships, leisure, and fun and the ability to stand up under pressure and tackle head-on challenges. Yet managing stress isn't one-size-fits-all. This is why experimenting and finding out what works best for you is important. There are numerous tips you can follow on how to handle the stress that will help in a rewarding way.

4.1 Know your routine

Let us define routine by looking into how impactful a routine can be from the world's finest, whose life looked like it was created in the best aspects of life. We've acquired horrendous know-how and put the expertise into the hands of our society's highly trained, highly skilled, and hardworking people. But that experience has burdened and protected us both. It has burdened us because there are just so many different things we have to do in a certain order, or we are going to fail. The amount is enormously growing.

But there is a way for us to deliver and use our knowledge safely, correctly, and reliably and by using a simple tool that has existed since the First Men. What builds routine. What a routine should be, and then?

Why it is important to follow a daily routine?

You might be familiar with the saying, "good is the enemy of great." And in many situations, it might seem like following a daily routine, and the schedule is just "good enough" by default. When you follow a routine, you lack the fun and spontaneity you need to be truly creative, right? Not quite. Our culture is already too full of spontaneity and passion for our own good.

The only way to do your utmost is to put in the time. Writers should write. Coders have to code.

You have to design the designers. This is getting harder to do, unfortunately. Social media, television, and news (not to mention "successful" distractions such as spending the whole day talking or emailing!)

 suck our attention away like vampires. On the other hand, achievement comes from hard work,

determination and a dedication even when you don't want to put in the work. As a behavioral scientist at Stanford, B. J.

Fogg wrote: When you select and order the right small actions, then you won't have to push yourself to make it grow. It just happens naturally, like a good seed planting in a good place.

Basically, in a number of ways, a routine benefits you:

Routines help you prioritize what counts. If you organize your day in a certain way or work hard to build clear habits, you essentially say, "this is what matters to me." Routines and habits cause you to think hard about your goals and make choices.

Understanding what you do every day helps remove distractions. As the best-selling author, Nir Eyal, says, "If you don't realize what you're distracted by, you can't say you're disturbed." When you've got a routine, you're more likely to notice when something's trying to take your attention away.

Habits free up energy for bigger tasks. The reason that 40 percent of our actions are driven by habit is that our minds love energy conservation. The more you can organize your daily activities, the more mental space and resources you need to participate in more important tasks.

Daily routines and habits are driving innovation — nothing like a creative muse. Instead, the most creative ideas come from constantly working and putting the effort in.

Routines and routines drive you forward. Your habits and routines are above all what makes you see change and inspire you to do more.

What is the difference between a habit and a routine?

A habit is a behavior or conduct that you have turned into an automatic response. You are stimulated by something (either externally as a message, or internally as a certain feeling), and you are compelled to follow it through.

On the other hand, a routine is a string of habits that you

develop for specific parts of the day. Perhaps it's a morning routine that you do when you wake up first. Or an afternoon routine to help you avoid the dip after lunch. We all have those habits, whatever it is. But we all don't know how powerful they are.

Why you can't just follow the successful everyday routine of famous developers and founders, if our lives and our progress rely on our routines and behaviors, then why not just follow other people's paths? Successful entrepreneurs and creatives love to chat about the way they spend their days and share their success "secrets." Yet simply trying to retrace their steps is a problem: Just because a procedure works for someone else, it doesn't mean it will work for you.

More than simply following the daily routines and behaviors of other people, the best way to become your best self is to challenge, explore and learn what works for you.

A routine can be a finely calibrated tool in the right hands to take advantage of a variety of limited resources: time the most limited resource of all, as well as determination, self-discipline and optimism. A solid routine encourages a well-worn rhythm for one's mental energy and helps stave off mood tyranny.

The big caveat here is that it's the routine that must suit the person doing it. We all have different triggers for behaviors, motivation levels and self-reliance on how we spend our time. And to say that you're exactly the same as someone like Elon Musk and can follow his routine is a catastrophe formula.

Alternatively, to maximize your own day, you need to experiment for yourself. More precisely, there are a few aspects of your life that you should look to build good habits and develop productive daily routines:

- Your morning routine

- Work habits to help you stay focused

- Disconnect from work

- Energy and health management

4.2 Find the source

Causes of Stress

Stress can come from many sources known as "stressors." Because our experience of what is considered "stressful" is generated by our individual interpretations of what we encounter in life (based on our own combination of personality traits, available resources, habitual thought patterns), one person can view a situation as "stressful" and just "challenging" by someone else.

Simply put, the stress trigger of one person may not register to someone else as stressful. That said, some situations in most people tend to cause more stress and may increase the burn out risk. For example, when we are in circumstances where there are high demands on us; where we have little power and few choices; where we don't feel equipped; where we can be harshly judged by others; and where there are severe or unexpected repercussions for failure, we tend to get stressed.

Because of this, their work, their relationships, their financial issues, health issues, and more mundane things like clutter or busy schedules stress many people. Learning skills to cope with these stressors will help lower your stress level.

Effects of Stress

Just as each of us perceives stress differently, stress affects us all in ways that are unique to us.

One person may experience headaches,

while another may find a common reaction to stomach upset, and one third may experience any of a number of other

symptoms. While we all respond to stress in our own ways, a long list of commonly experienced stress-related effects ranges from mild to life-threatening. Stress can have an effect on immunity, which can affect nearly all health areas. Stress can also affect mood in a number of ways.

When you have physical symptoms that you think may be related to stress, talk with your doctor to make sure you do what you can to protect your health. Symptoms that may be compounded by stress aren't "all in your mind," and they need to be treated. Developing a stress management plan is often one part of the overall wellness plan.

Identifying the various sources of stress in your life

Managing stress begins by recognizing the causes of stress in your life. That is certainly not as simple as it sounds. Although recognizing major stressors such as changing jobs, moving, or going through a divorce is easy, it may be more difficult to identify the causes of chronic stress. Overlooking how your own emotions, feelings, and habits lead to your daily stress levels is all too easy. Yeah, you may know you're constantly worried about work deadlines, but maybe it's your procrastination that causes stress, rather than the actual job demands.

Look closely at your routines, behaviors, and excuses to find the true causes of stress:

• Would you explain away stress as temporary ("I have about millions of things going on for now") as even though you can't remember the last time you took a proper breath?

• Would you define stress as an integral part of your routine life (' Things are always crazy around here') or as a part of your personality (' I have a lot of nervous energy, that's all')?

• Do you blame other persons or outside events for your tension, or do you perceive it as completely normal and unusual?

Your stress level will remain beyond your control until you accept responsibility for the part you play in generating or sustaining it.

How about a Journal of Stress? A stress journal will help you identify the stressors that are normal in your life and how you cope with them. Keep track of this in your journal each time you feel overwhelmed. You will start looking at trends and popular themes as you keep a daily log.

• What actually caused your stress (try to make a guess if you're uncertain)

• How you felt, both physically and emotionally

- How you responded

- What you did to make you relax and feel good.

Look at how you deal with stress

Talk about the ways you are currently managing your life and dealing with stress. Your journal of stress will help you identify these. Are your methods for coping safe or bad, effective or unproductive? Unfortunately, many people are dealing with stress in ways that compound the problem.

Unhealthy approaches to handle stress

These coping strategies can temporarily reduce stress, but in the long run, they cause more damage:

- Smoking extensively

- Drinking way too much

- Overeating or starving

- Zoning out for longer spans in front of the electronic media

- Withdrawal from friends, family, and activities

- Using pills or drugs to relax

- Too much sleep

- Procrastinating quite often

- Finding ways every minute of the day to avoid issues

- Releasing your aggression on others (lashing out, angry outbursts, physical violence)

Learning healthier ways to manage stress

If your stress management mechanisms don't lead to your improved physical and emotional health, it's time to find better ones. There are many healthy ways to cope with stress, but they all need to change. You can change the situation or change your answer. It's helpful to think of the four A's when determining which choice to choose: avoid, alter, adapt, or accept. Since everyone has a specific response to stress, there is no answer "one size fits all" to handle it. No single method works in any situation or for everyone, so play with different techniques and strategies. Reflect on what's keeping you calm and in control.

Dealing with Stressful Situations mainly includes

Change the very situation by simply,

- Avoid the stressor.

- Alter the stressor

Change your sudden or delayed reaction by,

- Adapt to the stressor.

- Accept the stressor.

4.3 Action plan

Action plan is a typical document that lists what steps need to be taken to achieve a specific objective. While there may seem nothing you can do about work and home stress,

 there are steps you can take to relieve the pressure and regain control.

An action plan seeks to explain what resources are needed to achieve the goal, to formulate a timetable for when certain activities need to be accomplished and to decide what resources are required.

Effective Stress Management

It might sound like you can do nothing about your stress level. The utility bills won't stop coming, there will never be more hours in the day for all your errands and there will always be overwhelming obligations for your job or family. But you have much more power than you'd expect. In reality, the simple awareness that you control your life is the basis for managing stress.

It's all about taking charge of managing stress: taking charge of your thoughts, emotions, schedule, environment, and how you dealt with the problems. The real ultimate goal is a balanced life, with time for work, relationships, relaxation, and fun plus the resilience to keep up under pressure and face challenges head-on.

Stress can be handled successfully in many different ways. The best stress reduction programs typically include a combination of stress relievers that cope physically and psychologically with stress and help develop resilience and coping skills.

Use rapid stress relievers. In just a few minutes, certain stress relief methods will help to relax the stress response of the body. Such strategies provide a "quick fix

" that helps you feel more calm right now, and this can help in a number of ways. You can address issues more thoughtfully and proactively if your stress response is not activated.

Out of frustration, you may be less likely to lash out at others, which may keep your relationships healthier.

 Nipping your stress response in your bud can also prevent you from suffering chronic stress.

Fast stress relievers such as breathing exercises may not develop your immunity to potential stress or reduce the stressors you face. Still, they can help calm the physiology of the body once the stress response is triggered.

Create habits that relieve stress. Many strategies are less effective when you're right in the middle of a stressful situation. But if you continuously practice them regularly, they can help you to overall cope with stress by being less reactive to it and more able to quickly and easily reverse your stress response. Long-term, healthy habits, such as exercise or daily meditation, will help promote stressor tolerance if you make them a routine part of your life. Communication skills and other lifestyle skills can help manage stressors and shift our emotions from being "overwhelmed" to being "challenged" or even "stimulated."

If possible, remove stressors. You may not be able to terminate stress entirely from your life or even the most significant stressors, but there are places where you can mitigate it and get it to a manageable level. Some stress you can relieve will reduce the overall stress load. For example, leaving only one toxic relationship will help you deal with other pressures you face more effectively because you may feel less stressed.

The exploration of a wide range of stress management strategies and then the option of a combination that matches your needs can be a key strategy for successful stress relief.

Stress Management Tips

People can learn to cope with stress and lead to healthier, happier lives. Here are some tips for keeping pressure at bay.

• Keep a right attitude.

• Understand that things are uncontrollable.

• Be assertive rather than aggressive. Instead of becoming angry, defensive, or passive, express your thoughts, views, or beliefs.

• Learn and practice relaxation techniques; try out stress management meditation, yoga, or tai-chi.

• Work out daily. The body is better able to combat stress when it's healthy.

• Eat well rounded, healthy meals.

• Know how to handle your time more effectively.

Correctly set boundaries and learn to say no to demands that would cause undue stress in your life.

• Take time to have hobbies, interests and relax.

• Get enough rest and get enough sleep as your body needs time to recover from stressful circumstances.

• To reduce stress, do not rely on alcohol, drugs or compulsive behaviors.

• To seek social support. Spend ample time with the ones you love.

• Get care with a psychologist or other mental health professional skilled in stress management or biofeedback strategies to learn healthy ways to cope with stress in your life.

Stress management strategy

#1: Avoid unnecessary stress

Not all stress can be avoided, and avoiding a situation that needs to be addressed isn't healthy. Nonetheless, you might be surprised by the number of stressors you can remove in your life.

Learn how to say "no"-Know and stick to your boundaries. Whether it is in your personal or professional life, simply refuse to accept additional responsibilities when you are close to reaching those responsibilities. Take on more than you can with the tension is a sure fire recipe.

Avoid people who stress you out–If someone in your life is continually causing stress and you can't turn the relationship around, reduce the amount of time you spend with that person or fully end the relationship.

Take control of your surroundings–If you're upset by the evening news, turn off the TV. If you are tensed with traffic, take a longer but less traveled route. If it's an unpleasant task to store, do your grocery shopping online.

Avoid hot-button subjects–Cross them off your discussion list if you're concerned about religion or politics. When you constantly disagree with the same people about the same thing, stop bringing it up or excuse yourself when it's the discussion topic.

Pare your to-do list–evaluate your schedule, obligations, and day-to-day work. If you are having too much on your plate, differentiate between the "shoulds" and the "musts." Remove activities that are not really important at the bottom of the list, or completely eliminate them.

#2: Alter the situation

If a difficult situation cannot be prevented, try to alter it. Find what you can do to change things so that the question doesn't show up in the future. This often involves changing how you communicate and how you work in your everyday life.

Instead of bottling them, share your thoughts. If you are disturbed by something or someone, express your thoughts freely and with respect. If you don't communicate your feelings, frustration will build up and the situation will probably stay the same.

Want to negotiate. When you expect someone to change their behavior, be prepared to do the same. If you're both willing to bend at least a little, you're going to have a good chance to find a happy middle ground.

Be assertive. Do not take your own life backseat. Tackle issues head-on, do your best to anticipate and prevent them. If you have an exam to prepare for and your chatty roommate just got home, tell them straight away that you only have five minutes to talk.

You better manage your time. Poor time management can cause considerable stress. It is hard to stay calm and focused when you're stretched too thin and running behind. But if you plan ahead of it and make sure you don't over-expand, you can change how much stress you're under.

#3: Adapt to the stressor

If you are unable to change the stressor, then change yourself. You can adapt to stressful situations by changing your expectations and attitude and regain your sense of control.

Problems with Reframe. Try to take a more positive view of stressful situations. Rather than complaining about a traffic jam, find it an excuse to stop and regroup, listen to your favorite radio station or enjoy some time alone.

Look at the picture big. Take the stressful situation into perspective. In the long run, ask yourself how important that will be. Will that matter in a month's time? One year? Is it worth getting upset over, really? If the answer is no, then focus your energy and resources elsewhere.

Set your standards. Perfectionism is a big source of stress that can be avoided. Stop setting yourself to failure by calling for perfection. Set reasonable expectations for yourself and others, and know "good enough" to be correct.

Concentrate on the positive. Take a moment alone to reflect on all the things you enjoy in your life when stress is getting you down, including your own positive qualities and gifts. This simple strategy will help you keep a perspective on things.

Adjusting your attitude by how you think your emotional and physical wellbeing can have a profound effect. Every time you think of yourself as a negative thought, your body reacts as if it were in the throes of a situation full of tension. You're more likely to feel confident when you see good things for yourself; the reverse is true, too. Eliminate terms like "ever," "never," "can," and "must." These are tale signs of self-defeating thoughts.

#4: Accept the things you can't change

Many causes of stress are imperative. You can't prevent or alter stressors like a loved one's death, a serious illness or a national recession. In such situations, acknowledging things as they are, is the only way to cope with tension. Acceptance can be tough, but it's better in the long run than protesting against a situation you can't alter.

Try not to control that which is uncontrollable. Some things in life are beyond our control— especially other people's behaviors. Focus on things you can control, such as how you choose to react to problems rather than stressing them.

Look upside down. As the saying goes, "What doesn't destroy us makes us stronger." Try to look at these as opportunities for personal growth when faced with major challenges. If your own poor choices have led to a stressful situation, think about them and learn from your mistakes.

Share your impressions. Speak to a trusted friend or arrange a rendezvous with a therapist. It can be very cathartic to describe what you are going through, even if there is nothing you can do to change the stressful situation.

Get to understand forgiveness. Accept the fact that we're living in an imperfect world and people are making mistakes. Let go of the resentments and rage. Through forgiving and moving on, free yourself from negative energy.

#5: Make time for fun and relaxation

You must minimize stress in your life by cultivating yourself beyond a take charge mentality and a positive attitude. When you regularly make time for fun and relaxation, when they arrive, eventually, you will be in a better place to handle the stressors of life.

Going for a walk, spending time in nature can be healthy ways to relax and refresh. You should call a good mate, or use a good workout to sweat out the stress. You can also write in your newspaper, take a long bath, light up scented candles, savor a warm cup of tea or coffee, play with a cat. Perhaps working in your yard and getting a massage. Sticking up with a good book or listening to music and watching a movie.

Don't get so lost in the hustle and bustle of life that you're unable to look after your own needs. Primary care is a requirement, not a privilege. Set aside time to rest. Include, in your daily schedule, rest and relaxation. Don't allow encroachment on other obligations. Take a detailed break from all duties and recharge your batteries.

Connect with people. Spend time with those positive people who make your life better. A strong system of support will shake you from the negative effects of stress. Do something that you love every single day. Whether it's stargazing, playing the piano or working on your bike, make time for leisure activities that bring you joy. Maintain your sense of humor. This includes the ability to self-laugh. The laughing act helps the body combat stress in a number of ways.

Learn to respond to relaxation. You can regulate the stress levels by relaxation techniques that activate the body's response to relaxation, a state of restfulness that is the opposite of the response to stress. Practicing these strategies on a regular basis will develop your physical and emotional strength, heal your body and improve your overall sense of joy and equanimity.

#6: Adopt a healthy lifestyle

Strengthening your physical health will improve your resilience to stress. Work out daily. Physical activity plays a key role in mitigating the negative effects and avoiding them. Allow an exercise time of at least 30 minutes, three days a week. None of this beats aerobic exercise to relieve pent-up energy and tension.

Eat good food. Well-nourished bodies are better suited to coping with stress, so be mindful of what you eat. Begin your day with breakfast and keep your energy and mind clear throughout the day with healthy, nutritious meals.

Reduce the amount of caffeine and sugar. Temporary "highs" of caffeine and sugar often lead to a mood and energy crash. You can feel more relaxed and sleep better by reducing the amount of coffee, soft drinks, candy and sugar snacks in your diet.

Avoid alcohol, drugs and cigarettes. Alcohol or substance self-medication can provide an easy way out of stress but the relief is only temporary. Do not avoid the problem at hand or disguise it; deal with issues head on and with a clear mind.

Get lots of sleep. Adequate sleep is fueling the mind and body. You'll feel tired because it can cause you to think irrationally.

Practice the 4 A's of stress management

Although the stress is a kind of automatic response from your nervous system, certain stressors come up at regular times: for example, your commute to work, a meeting with your boss, or family reunions. One way you can either change the situation or change the response if you treat these predictable stressors. It's helpful to think about the four A's when determining which choice to choose in any given scenario: avoid, alter, adapt, or accept.

Avoid unnecessary stress

Avoiding a stressful situation that needs to be addressed is not safe, but you may be surprised by the number of stressors you may remove in your life.

Learn how to say "no." Learn and stick to your boundaries. Whether you are in your personal or professional life, taking on more than you can handle is a recipe for stress, which is surefire. Just distinguish between the "shoulds" and the "musts" and tell "no" to take on too much where possible.

Evite the people who stress you out. If someone causes stress regularly in your life, limit the amount of time you spend with that person or terminate the relationship.

Take the power of your environment. If you get nervous about the evening news, turn off the TV. Take a longer but less-traveled path if traffic makes you nervous. If it's an unpleasant chore to go to the store, do your grocery shopping online.

Check your list of to-dos. Analyze your schedule, your duties and your everyday tasks. When you have too much on your plate, drop tasks that are not really needed at the bottom of the list or completely eliminate them.

Alter the situation

When you can't escape a stressful situation, try to change it. This often involves changing how you communicate and how you work in your everyday life.

Share your emotions rather than bottle them up. If you are upset by something or someone, be more assertive and express your thoughts freely and with respect. If you have an exam to prepare for and your chatty roommate just got home, tell them right up front that you have only five minutes to talk. If you don't share your emotions, there will be anger and tension.

Want to compromise When you expect someone to change their behavior, be prepared to do the same. If you're both willing to bend at least a little, there's a good chance you'll reach a happy middle ground.

Create a timetable that is balanced. All the work, and no play, is a burnout recipe. Try to find a balance or manage between work and family life, social and solitary tasks, day-to-day commitments and downtime.

Adapt to the stressor

If you are unable to change the stressor, then change yourself. You can respond to stressful situations by adjusting your perceptions and attitude and recover your sense of control.

Problems with Reframe. Try to take a more positive view of the stressful situations. Instead of fuming about a traffic jam, look at it as an excuse to pause and reassemble, listen to your favorite radio station, or enjoy some time alone.

Look at the picture big. Take the stressful situation into perspective. In the long run, ask yourself how important that will be. Is that going to matter in a month? One year? Is it worth getting upset over, really? If the answer is No, focus your energy and resources elsewhere.

Customize the expectations. The perfectionism is a big source of stress that can be avoided. Stop setting up by demanding perfection for failure. Set the reasonable expectations for yourself and others, and learn to be OK with "good enough." Take a moment alone to reflect on all the things you enjoy in your life when stress is getting you down, including your own positive qualities and gifts. This simple strategy will help you keep a perspective on things.

Accept the things you can't change

Those causes of stress are inevitable.

You can't prevent or alter stressors like a loved one's death, a serious illness or a national recession. In such situations, acknowledging things as they are being the only way to cope with tension. Acceptance can be challenging, but it's better in the long run than protesting against a situation that you can't change.

Seek not to govern that which is uncontrollable. Some things in life are beyond our control, particularly other people's behaviors. Reflect on things you can control, such as how you choose to respond to problems, rather than stressing them.

Look upside down. Try to look at these as opportunities for personal growth while facing major obstacles. If your own poor choices have led to a stressful situation, think about them and learn from your errors.

Learn to pardon. Understand that we are living in an imperfect world and people are making mistakes. Let go of resentment and anger. Through forgiving and moving on, free yourself from negative energy.

Share the feelings. It can be very cathartic to share what you are going through, even if there is nothing you can do to improve the stressful situation. Speak to a trusted friend or arrange a meeting with a therapist.

Few More Tips

Tip 1: Get moving

The last thing you're likely to feel like doing when you're depressed is getting up and exercising. Yet physical activity is a major relief of stress— and in order to experience the benefits you don't have to be an athlete or spend hours in a gym. Exercises works on releasing endorphins that make you feel good and can also be a valuable distraction from your everyday concerns.

While you will get the most gain from exercising regularly for 30 minutes or more, gradually building up your fitness level is OK. Even very small things will add up in a day. The first step is to get up and on the move. Here are some easy ways to integrate exercise into your daily schedule:

• Put on some music and dance around

• Take your dog for a stroll

• Walk or cycle to the grocery store

• Use the stairs at home or work instead of an elevator

• Park your car at the farthest spot in the lot and walk the rest of the way

• Join your workout partner and motivate each other as you work out

• Play ping-pons

The stress-busting magic of careful rhythmic exercises is important. Although virtually any form of physical activity can help to burn off tension and stress, rhythmic exercises are particularly effective. Walking, biking, swimming, dancing, spinning, tai chi and aerobics are all good choices. But whatever you choose, make sure you enjoy it so you're more likely to stick to it.

Make a conscious effort while you are exercising to pay attention to your body and the physical (and sometimes emotional) sensations you feel when you walk. For example, focus on matching your breathing with your actions, or note how the air or sunlight on your skin feels. Adding this dimension of mindfulness will help you break the cycle of negative thoughts that often accompany overwhelming stress.

Tip 2: Connect to others

Nothing is more relaxing than to spend quality time with

another human being that makes you feel comfortable and understandable. Apparently, face-to-face contact activates a cascade of hormones that counteracts the body's defensive response to "fight-or-flight." It is one of the greatest source of stress in nature (as an added bonus it also helps to stave off depression and anxiety). And make sure you communicate frequently-and in person-with your family and friends.

Keep in mind that you don't need to be able to fix the depression on the people you talk to. We have got to be good listeners. So try not to let fears about appearing weak or being a burden discourage you from opening up. The people you care about will be flattered by your confidence. It just strengthens the bond.

Of course, it is not always realistic to have a pal close by to lean on when you feel overwhelmed by stress, but you can improve your resilience to life's stressors by building and maintaining a network of close friends.

There are some tips for building good relationships

1. Help out a colleague at work

2. Try to Help or guide someone else by volunteering

3. Share a lunch or snack with a close one

4. Ask a close one to check or monitor you regularly

5. Accompany any of your friends or someone to the movies or a concert

6. Contact an old friend

7. Prefer a walk with a workout buddy

8. Plan a weekly or monthly dinner or lunch date

9. Befriends with new people by taking a new root towards different activities

10. Always confide in a clergy member, mentor, teacher, or sports coach

Tip 3: Make time for fun and relaxation

You will alleviate stress in your life by leveraging "me" time beyond a take-up approach and a positive attitude. Don't get so lost in the hustle and bustle of life that you're unable to look after your own needs. Primary care is a necessity, not a privilege. When you regularly make time to have fun and relax, you'll be in a great place to handle the stressors of life.

Set some leisure time aside. Include, in your daily schedule, rest and relaxation. Don't allow encroachment on other obligations. Make up your mind that now this is your time to take a break and recharge your batteries.

Do something that you love every single day. Whether it's stargazing, playing the piano or working on your bike, make time for leisure activities that bring you joy.

Maintain your sense of humor. This includes the ability to self laugh. The laughing act helps your body combat stress in a number of ways.

Come up with a calming drill. There are some relaxation techniques such as yoga, meditation, and deep breathing that stimulate the body's response to relaxation, a state of restfulness that is the opposite of the reaction to battle or flight or tension mobilization. When you study and practice these methods, your stress levels drop and your mind and body become relaxed and concentrated.

Tip 4: Manage your time better

Poor time management can cause considerable stress. It is hard to stay calm and focused when you're stretched too thin and running behind.

Plus, you'll be tempted to stop or minimize all the healthy things you're supposed to do to keep tension in check, such as socializing occasionally and getting enough sleep. The best news is that there are things you can do to strike a better balance between work and life.

Don't make over-commitments. Do not schedule things back-to-back or try to fit too much into a single day. All too often, we underestimate the amount of time it will take.

Place activities first. Make a list of the activities you need to perform and answer them in order of importance. Next, do the high priority things. If you have something to do that is particularly unpleasant or frustrating, get it over with early. As a result, the remainder of your day will be more pleasant.

Projects split into small steps. If a big project seems daunting, do a step-by-step plan. Reflect on one easy step at a time, instead of taking on everything at once.

Responsibility Delegate. You just don't have to take the pressure of doing it all by yourself, be it at home, at school or at work. If other people are able to take care of that mission, why not let them? Let go of the will to monitor or supervise every small step. In the meantime, you'll let go of unnecessary stress.

Tip 5: Maintain balance with a healthy lifestyle

There are other healthy lifestyle options in addition to regular exercise that can increase the resistance to stress.

Eat a good diet. Well-nourished bodies are better prepared for pain, so be mindful of what you are eating. Begin your day with breakfast and keep your energy and mind clear throughout the day with healthy, nutritious meals.

Reduce sugar and caffeine. Temporary "highs" of caffeine and sugar often contribute to a mood and energy crash. By reducing your diet's amount of coffee, soft drinks, chocolate, and sugary snacks, you'll feel more relaxed and sleep better.

Avoid drugs, cigarettes and alcohol.

Alcohol or drug self-medication can provide an easy way out of stress but the relief is only temporary. Do not avoid the problem at hand or disguise it; deal with issues head on and with a clear mind.

Get lots of sleep. Adequate amount of sleep is fueling the mind and the whole body. If you are feeling tired, it will increase your stress because it can cause irrational thinking.

Tip 6: Learn to relieve stress at the moment

You just need a way to manage your stress levels right now when you're frazzled by your morning commute, trapped in a tense meeting at work, or fried out of another argument with your partner. This is where the relief from swift stress comes in.

The best way to reduce tension is to take a deep breath and use what you see, hear, taste, and touch with your senses or through a calming movement. By watching a favorite photo, smelling a particular scent, listening to a favorite piece of music, degusting a piece of gum or, for example, embracing a pet, you can relax easily and concentrate on yourself. Not everyone, of course, reacts equally to every sensory experience. Experimenting and finding the special sensory experiences that work best for you.

4.4 A new beginning

Wouldn't it be really great to know what your wellbeing will have in the future? We could see our aging selves and any health problems we would end up with if we had a crystal ball. The truth is, we live longer, but we don't live healthier.

Live a better quality of life.

The Quality of Life should not be confused with the idea of living standards, which is mainly based on income. Alternatively, normative quality of life metrics includes not only wealth and employment but also the built environment, physical and mental health, schooling, recreation, and leisure and social association.

One has to realize that the best idea is to leave the world while walking on your feet. The secret to that is confidence. One woman is giving birth. An addict pours his booze bottle over the drain. A worker is an overseer. In a car accident, a daughter loses her mother. New beginnings will occur at any time of day. Often, however, new beginnings might not be our own choice or our own taste. The worker may not have predicted the promotion or desired it. On the other hand, the addict has made a clear choice to try out a different path indicated by the dumping of his precious liquor. We are both entering a time of new beginnings. And although a child's birth and a loved one's death seem very different, they both have two things in common: an end and a beginning.

Walking through the threshold of a new season of existence can be appallingly challenging. How do we live effectively in the midst of a new beginning we had not anticipated or even wanted? What can we do to glorify God if our situations are not just new but also extremely painful? Each time we let something old go, there's discomfort, even pain. We encounter a great sense of loss, even hopelessness, whenever we lose something or somebody of great importance. Yet it is comforting to remember that the seemingly greatest loss of all, the death of Jesus, resulted in a resurrected Christ's best new beginning ever.

The new beginning and new life allow us to live our lives to the fullest, whatever we may have missed or let go of, for we are never alone in God.

We are cherished forever.

We can always trust God to deliver the best.

He sees far beyond our pain and suffering and if we let him, he has a way to make any new beginning good for us and those around us. We will succeed through this cycle and even find peace and joy in the midst of letting go.

All these habits and tips will help you make yourself more successful. But it is probably a bad idea to try to add them all to your daily routine. You need to try instead and see what works for you. Try one for a week and follow up with the tests. Is it working? Why didn't they?

Eventually, we will always do what works best for us, by necessity. If certain things aren't working for you, your body and mind will tell you (you'll get restless, depressed, nervous, tired, etc...). Hear these signs and use them to create your own personalized daily routine.

The best way to experience a new beginning is to follow the concept of Lean On God

Live in the truth

Whether you're battling a tempting addiction or mourning an untimely loss, remaining rooted in God's Word of truth is a key to accepting any new beginning. We are prone to fall victim to lies that increase our pain and keep us from increasing and moving forward without a base of truth.

Enlist others for support

In the safety net of caring and competent Religious friend's new beginnings are best confronted. God is a relational individual. Jesus had not been a lone ranger. His inner circle of followers encircled him. We will also find support, motivation, and assistance from others who have experienced similar circumstances.

Approach God boldly

We have a great opportunity to approach our holiness with boldness and confidence.

David gave us the perfect example in the psalms of how to reach out to God in every conceivable way, even in our wrath, our sorrow, and our anxiety. Without the grace of God, we do not need to face anything. We can go confidently to him because he asks us that we can.

Never give up

No matter what our present circumstances can look like, no matter how difficult it might be to let go, we win in the end with God. It may seem we are losing, but in the end, goodness and glory will flourish in the midst of a new start. We just simply need to keep our eyes on our leader and put one foot in front of the other before we cross the finish line.

Overcome obstacles

When we're in the midst of letting go, we may find ourselves burdened by a barrage of barriers on our road that can prevent us from going through tomorrow's door of a better life. Grief and heartache emotions can be part of the new start process. Lingering negative thoughts and feelings can become barriers that hold us trapped. With the grace of God and the love of others, we can go forward, get rid of everything that holds us back.

Neutralize the enemy

It's very clear from the various Holy books that Religious people have an enemy. This enemy of our souls wants to destroy us and keep us from embracing the purpose of God for our lives. By using the armor that God so kindly offers, we will kill this beast. Carry on the shield every day.

Go forward with God

This is much like "don't give up." New beginnings can be daunting, and we can be frozen, scared to take another step. We need not carry on with our own resources. In reality, our limited human capacity isn't going to be enough, but all things are possible with God. Let him lead, as you lean upon him.

Open your eyes

Look at the beauty that surrounds you on your journeys. Once you embrace your new beginning, you will discover the wonderful ways in which God works inside you and around you. And in your darkest hour, God is there. You can see his light if you look.

Decide to worship

We thank God, in any case, brings benefits far beyond our highest expectations. If we achieve liberation from slavery or addiction, it is only natural that our Deliverer should be praised. Yet worship may seem out of place when a new beginning is the product of failure. And imagine Paul, in his jail cell, praising God. Worship touches God's very heart, and in exchange, it touches ours. Worship God, and look to the best.

Depend on Him, and expect a glorious new start after another. We can be filled with the strength of the Holy Spirit every new day that will aid us in our new beginnings.

Not knowing is what's best

1. Not knowing takes the pressure off.

We get stressed out when we think we should learn when we don't know things. But when we see that our natural state is not knowing, we can actually open ourselves into that, into a state of curious detachment, childlike wonder. Which will happen next? Will that be a pleasant surprise, an opportunity to know, or both?

We can see that we do not know anything, in a sense. We never knew anything about it. So we're just giving it our best shot when the time comes to make a decision. So we know that if we need to change.

2. Not knowing saves time.

You look at the world differently,

because you think you don't guess (and can't know). Think of the time and money we waste trying to predict the future. I'm an ardent sports radio fan. Around ninety percent of this is pure speculation about who will gain or who will lose and what that really means. And the answer is no different, like the debt crisis, the economy, or the next race for the presidency.

We do not know what will happen to any of this stuff. I just believe it is valid. Rather than trying to keep up with what all the pundits say, we should spend our time doing things that we love, including spending time with our spouse and children. Or just have a walk in the park.

3. Not knowing fosters learning.

If I had known the outcome, I wouldn't have taken up my current career. And in the end, I'd missed it so much. I truly believe we can all point to bad experiences we wouldn't have chosen — a hard job, the loss of someone near us, coping with a health problem.

And yet the majority of our development stems from suffering. I witnessed paraplegics and victims of cancer smile as they describe the development that came from their illness, insisting that they wouldn't have anything else. Sometimes we remember just in retrospect how important an experience was.

4. Not knowing brings the joy of surprise.

Of course, we don't want to know when there will be bad stuff. But what about one friend's surprise call? What was part of the windfall you didn't know? What about a child laughing?

A lot of lasting happiness always comes from surprise. And knowing exactly what is to come would take away all of that.

5. We have no choice.

Let's face it. the natural state of things is not understanding. When we want to know things we can't know (like the future, or the best course of action), all we build for ourselves is a disappointment. I know it may sound like "suck it up, you can't change anything," but we can change a lot, really. Once we realize that what happens can not be managed, we can devote more of our time to how we react and what we know. And in the process, we will open ourselves to a new sense of ease.

5. Conclusion

Boosting your health appears to be more challenging while being stuck in the grasp of unhealthiness. A healthy lifestyle seems to be a primary concern of most of the people these days. The modern world we live in has advanced in so many ways, and it is essential to learn and follow all the parameters regarding healthy living. These dynamic standards are linked with anything we eat or anyone we interact with. More recently, there have been researches that define health as a body's ability to adapt to new threats and illnesses. The idea originating from this is; in recent decades, modern science has dramatically increased human awareness of diseases and how they work. Both mental and physical forms are often discussed. There are so many lifestyle habits dealing with those issues that can go a long way in improving the chances of a long and healthy life. Life is much more than good health, and it equally involves social and spiritual wellbeing. Healthy diet and stress management, diving into a passion or hobby and sometimes tapping on your back yourself should be high on your priority. It is an understanding that poor habits are hard to break, so you won't regret this decision until you follow a healthier lifestyle. Healthy habits reduce the risk of weak health, and improve your overall appearance and mental health, and results in a much-needed boost to your energy level. It is hard for a person to change attitude and routine immediately, but one step at a time is pretty much helpful.

Unhealthiness is debated in relation to the life cycle and society. The overall emphasis on root causes that are closely linked to poor health standards are highlighted under the circumstances that people are born with. Moreover, the social determinants playing their role for unhealthiness are developed under the concept of livelihood, customs, and distribution of wealth, power, and resources at global, regional, and local levels. These factors are described as the ones contributing more to the current state of health of an individual in all possible ways.

One must make sure that the grocery list contains as many healthy foods as possible. You will easily find that all the healthy foods and herbs have something in common. They have ingredients, like grain, fruit, vegetable, or dairy products. It is always advised to carefully observe the ingredients, for example, are they organic or plant-based. With this, you are always able to find yourself in good shape of your health. Along with the consumption of different foods, herbs and spices have been incredibly important. Before their culinary use, they are accepted for their medicinal properties. Modern day science has shown us that there are significant health benefits of them. With such natural treasures, a well-balanced diet plan offers all the energy you require to stay active throughout the day, plus the balanced and scheduled use of nutrients helps you to develop and repair your body and assist you in staying active and healthy and help you prevent diet-related diseases. It has been proven that maintaining and eating a healthy, balanced diet can help you stay healthy. This will affirmatively inspire you to change your health and take a closer look at what you eat.

Understanding the biggest struggle to manage health was to discover how to manage stress. Stress response of our body is a concern if it continuously suggests danger over problems that aren't there in the first place. Stress management helps you to adapt to your mind and body (resilience). Your body could always be on a high alert, without it. Stress can lead to severe health problems over time. Before stress affects your health, relationships, or quality of life, don't take any chances. From today, start practicing stress management strategies and simply understand that we are living in an imperfect world where no one is perfect. Just let go of resentment and anger through forgiving and moving on. Free yourself from all kinds of negative energy. You need to understand that the best idea is to leave the world, leaving good memories and, most importantly, walking on your feet. In the end, we will always do what actually works best for us. There are things that aren't working for you; your intuition will let you know. Observe these signs and attributes and make sure you strategize them to create your own personalized healthy routine. Anyone can go into a win-win situation by following a healthy routine. And certainly, anyone who believes in being healthy always finds a way to get over an unhealthy lifestyle.

6. References

Health benefits Retrieved from **https://www.medicalnewstoday.com/articles/150999.php**.

6 Positive Lifestyle Factors That Promote Good Health. (2020). Retrieved from https://www.verywellhealth.com/lifestyle-factors-health-longevity-prevent-death-1132391

A-Z of the root causes of ill health by Public Health England on Exposure. (2020). Retrieved from **https://publichealthengland.exposure.co/az-of-the-root-causes-of-ill-health**

5 Benefits of Healthy Habits. (2020). Retrieved from **https://www.healthline.com/health/5-benefits-healthy-habits#takeaway**

10 Delicious Herbs and Spices With Powerful Health Benefits. (2020). Retrieved from **https://www.healthline.com/nutrition/10-healthy-herbs-and-spices**

Why Stress Management Is So Important for Your Health. (2020). Retrieved from **https://www.mindbodygreen.com/0-2557/Why-Stress-Management-Is-So-Important-for-Your-Health.html**

Robinson, L. (2020). Stress Management. Retrieved from **https://www.helpguide.org/articles/stress/stress-management.htm**

Stress Management: How to Reduce, Prevent, and Cope with Stress. (n.d.). Retrieved from **https://www.brainline.org/article/stress-management-how-reduce-prevent-and-cope-stress**

What Is Stress Management? . Retrieved from **https://www.heart.org/en/healthy-living/healthy-lifestyle/stress-management/what-is-stress-management**

Gunnars, K. 5 Diets That Are Supported by Science. Retrieved from **https://www.healthline.com/nutrition/meal-plans**

www.ingramcontent.com/pod-product-compliance
Lightning Source LLC
Chambersburg PA
CBHW070715250726
48662CB00001B/430